# NOT GOING GENTLY

## A PSYCHOLOGIST FIGHTS BACK AGAINST ALZHEIMER'S FOR HER MOTHER...AND PERHAPS HERSELF

## by CONSTANCE L. VINCENT, PhD

ISBN: 1499512597
ISBN-13: 9781499512595
Library of Congress Control Number: 2014913022
CreateSpace Independent Publishing Platform
North Charleston, South Carolina

# DEDICATION

*To Madeline, my mother, whose love and strength continue to inspire me, and to all individuals and their families who face the challenge of dementia.*

# NOT GOING GENTLY

## TABLE OF CONTENTS

# PREFACE

When my mother first began to show signs of memory loss, I thought she only needed to try harder to concentrate, to focus and pay attention to conversations so she could remember what was being said. Then as my father showed increasing cognitive decline in his last years, I assumed it was a delayed effect of the lack of oxygen to his brain during the two open-heart surgeries he'd undergone. In short, I was in denial and wouldn't recognize even the possibility of Alzheimer's disease in either of the parents I loved.

My interest, as a developmental psychologist, was on a healthy, successful passage through all the stages of life—in short, on normal development, even if "normal" might be a little unconventional. I left neuroses, psychoses, and other deviant conditions to the field of abnormal psychology. I wanted to investigate change in its most positive forms—that is, the ways in which people can continue to grow intellectually, socially, and emotionally throughout life, adding rich experiences and depths of insight as the years go by.

The classes I taught at the university level reflected my own chronological age and changes. While my children were young, my class load was primarily filled with child psychology classes. As they and I grew older, I taught classes in adolescent and adult development. Finally, I taught Psychology of Aging, when I was in late middle age. I was still young and optimistic enough to focus on all of the positive aspects age could bring: the accumulation of wisdom, the wealth of life memories, the understanding and tolerance gained by experience. I emphasized the plasticity of the brain and its ability to continue to learn and form new neurons well into old age as evidenced by the most successful nonagenarians, some of whom came to my classes as inspirational guest speakers.

My students were encouraged, or rather, assigned, to find individuals who were able to remain active and engaged well into their later years. This wasn't such a difficult assignment; one study of thirty-two New Englander super-centenarians found that 89 percent were still living independently at age 93, and a startling 35 percent were independent at age 102.1 Indeed, my students succeeded in interviewing a number of amazing people, sometimes their own grandparents, whom they now viewed with greater appreciation. Of course, I wasn't naïve enough to ignore that with age there are also losses as well as some disappointments and regrets. But the goal of aging according to many psychologists, Carl Jung and Erik Erikson among them, is to incorporate all of life's experiences into a meaningful whole, to find integrity and not despair. I hoped my students would come away from the class with the same view I held—that aging could be the capstone of a life well lived.

Alzheimer's disease (AD) had no place in my view of aging. In fact, it has no place in anyone's view of normal aging. Alzheimer's is well known to be a terrible disease, unlike the ordinary, small memory losses that may accompany age. The disease eventually ravages so much more than memory: AD destroys one's ability to think and reason, to take care of one's own personal needs, and eventually to recognize one's own family. And it strikes indiscriminately.

Whether or not the dementia my father suffered in his last few years was late-onset Alzheimer's disease, vascular dementia, or a combination of mixed dementias, we'll never know for sure. Dad had had two open-heart surgeries: bypass and valve replacement. Research indicates that about half the patients who have such surgeries experience a later cognitive decline because the reduction in the blood flow of oxygen may damage the brain.[2]

Dad certainly had some form of dementia, a general term often defined as "a cognitive decline severe enough to interfere with daily life." Once, when he was almost eighty, my very intelligent father confided to me his fear that he could no longer "call the shots," an expression of his I'd never liked, but I knew what he meant. It was true he'd begun to show signs of what he called "slowing down." He used to chide my Aunt Mary for saying that about herself; my father would point out the self-fulfilling prophecy. "And every time she said it, she got slower and slower," he'd say. Now it was his turn.

When Dad's symptoms first became noticeable to others, he seemed to have difficulty following the plots of movies and television. Then it was the newspaper, his favorite thing to read, that he had trouble understanding; finally, in the mornings my mother used to sit next to him on the sofa and read the daily paper to him. Next he became disoriented and couldn't find his way around my house when he visited; apparently he'd lost the sense of spatial navigation related to the parietal lobes (no wonder he and my mother later became lost in the desert). Once, in a fast-food restaurant, he couldn't pay for the sandwich he'd ordered. Instead, he handed me his wallet and, with a pathetic look, pleaded, "You do it. I can't." For years, due to arthritis, he also had suffered bone-on-bone knee pain, but my brother, Michael, a medical doctor no doubt worried about further surgery complications, stopped him from getting a knee replacement, saying he'd had enough operations. Other family members or doctors weren't involved in this decision, one that my father lived to regret.

Dad's mental abilities quite rapidly declined, even more after he broke his hip and went to live in a rehabilitation center the last four months of his life. During that period, my husband Ed and I traveled to Nevada to visit him on two separate occasions. The second visit was early in December, just before Dad's eighty-seventh birthday. At that time he seemed more confused than on our previous visit, but he certainly still recognized Ed and me and talked clearly and rationally with us, although he appeared to be very depressed and broken hearted. I offered to tune his radio for him to the kind of big band music that he enjoyed, hoping it might cheer him a little, but he made a face and a dismissive motion with his hands as if to say it was useless now, so why bother? Once he'd realized he wouldn't be allowed to leave that facility and return to my brother's home, he apparently gave up all hope and desire to live. When we hugged good-bye, I had the feeling I might never see him again. Sadly, I was correct.

My sister Kate described visiting him two weeks later on Christmas Eve, always our Dad's favorite night of the year. The group of relatives with Kate included her husband, my mother and brother, and a cousin, all on their way to my cousin's house for a dinner party featuring the holiday Italian dishes my father loved to prepare and eat. Kate said Dad was then in such a poor condition they couldn't even contemplate taking him in a wheelchair to the party. His rapid failing since our last visit would indicate that he perhaps had had a stroke in the interim. He died nine days later, on January 2, 2005.

At the time my father, Michael, passed away, my mother, Madeline, was already showing signs of mild cognitive impairment, called MCI, a stage between normal aging changes and mild dementia. Her memory was noticeably affected, but she was still able to independently perform the basic activities of daily living. I was determined to keep my mother from ever joining the group whose MCI advanced to Alzheimer's disease.

Mom had always been my good friend, my confidant. As the oldest child, I was her often-reluctant helper, but now I have fond memories of working alongside her. Like many women of the 1950s, she was a housewife—the family caretaker whose days were filled with physical chores. Before pre-prepared foods, I helped her can tomatoes and other vegetables from our garden each autumn. Before automatic appliances, we pulled sheets through a wringer washer and scurried to gather drying clothes off the clothesline when sudden summer rains began to fall. Before permanent-press clothes, I came home from school each Tuesday (she was that scheduled) to the smell of starched and freshly ironed clothes. She excelled at all of the homemaking activities, especially cooking. Everyone in the extended family on my father's side wanted to eat the special dishes Aunt Lee (her nickname) brought to family picnics. Even her simple potato salad was justly famous, and the recipe was passed around.

But she wasn't all work all the time. Mom could be fun and laughter, playing badminton outside with us in the summer, teaching us to dance the polka to one of the polka bands on the radio Sunday afternoons while dinner was cooking and my father read the Sunday paper. We were ready for the German-Croatian weddings her side of the family had in big halls, where we danced the polka, but also slid in our stocking feet with the other cousins over sawdust covered floors. Mom and I listened to radio programs together before we got our first small black-and-white television set in 1953; the Saturday afternoon shows like *A Date with Judy* were our favorites—unless I was going to a movie with my friends. (Two dimes covered admission and a five-cent box of Milk Duds).

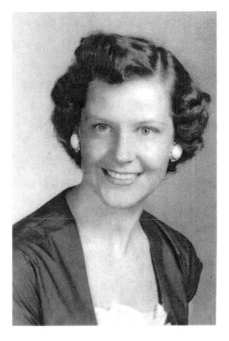

*Madeline in her mid-thirties, around 1955*

My parents never owned more than one car at a time, and my mother didn't learn to drive until I was in junior high school, just a few years before she taught me to drive. We both had the same problems with the standard transmission on our Plymouth, but I had the benefit of her experiences when she forgot to release the hand brake, especially the time she jerked the car down the street in front of everyone after church one Sunday. We laughed later, but neither of us ever wanted that ridicule again. Fortunately, my father traded in the Plymouth for a Buick with automatic transmission.

From the time I was in junior high school, Mom made many of the clothes for her self, my sisters, and me. Her father had been a tailor, and somehow my mother had absorbed his skill. She made coats and suits as well as dresses and skirts, some with very intricate detailing. Mom and I spent many an hour together in fabric stores, searching for a pattern we liked and the material that would do it justice. It wasn't unusual for us to come home with a yard of material and a zipper, then sew a skirt for me to wear that evening. Even after I moved to California in 1966, she continued to sew for my older daughter Karen and me, using our measurements and sending from Pennsylvania beautiful, perfectly fitting clothes (sometimes with a matching outfit for one of Karen's dolls). After cutting out patterns became too difficult for her, she learned to knit instead of sew. She made a sweater for me and lovely afghan throws for all of us. (Sadly, in her new residence, she didn't have even one afghan left to cover her when she took a nap until I bought one for her.)

For my mother's seventy-fifth birthday, we siblings had a big party for her at the country club where Kate and her husband George were members. When it was my turn to toast Mom, I referred to the recent Academy Awards and pointed out that if Oscars were given for best mother, choosing just one category to describe our mother's many skills would be really difficult.

What could we do to help her? Were we already too late? I began to study and read as much as I could about dementia and Alzheimer's disease in order to learn the best diet, the best supplements, and the best activities that would help save my mother. I was ready to fight back. And if I couldn't completely protect her from eventual AD, I at least wanted her to be active and healthy, enjoying her present life, for as long as possible.

My task was complicated, however, by two rather serious obstacles. First, since I live near San Francisco and my mother was then living near Las Vegas, we were separated by either a long, nine-hour drive or an airplane flight. Second, I had no legal control over where she'd live or over her care, as my brother administered her affairs. Other than the trips I'd take to visit her, or the times I'd arrange for her to come and stay with me, I had to rely on telephone calls in order to keep regular contact with her. I began a habit of calling her a few times a week before she went to bed, mainly to keep her mind stimulated with conversation and her spirits up by wishing her good night with a hug and kiss over the phone. But as time went on and she was moved from living with my brother in his home to being placed into care facilities, her side of the conversation became more emotional, full of fears and her hopes of escape. I started to record her statements because they were profoundly sad, coming from the depths of her feelings as she struggled to understand her new environments. Her words and her predicament touched me deeply, and I was totally frustrated at being legally powerless to intervene.

Clearly, Mom's memory losses were becoming worse. She was lonely, living apart from her family, and lacking mental as well as social stimulation on any regular basis. As you'll read, two dramatic incidents in particular exacerbated and hastened her decline. Although my original notes of our conversations were for my own journal and not intended for a book, I decided to tell my mother's story. Beyond the events in her life, I also wanted to summarize what I was learning about AD in my efforts to help her.

Two of the facts I discovered affected me personally. First, almost two out of every three Alzheimer's patients are female. Second, the chance of developing Alzheimer's may be higher if a person's mother had the disease. My manuscript began to follow the overlapping stories of my mother's decline and my own early memory losses that are due, I still hope, to normal aging. My research followed the path from common age-related memory problems to the early signs of dementia in mild cognitive impairment and then on to AD itself.

Of the sources I consulted, two were especially helpful. The Johns Hopkins publications have been invaluable, particularly the books written or edited by Peter V. Rabins, MD, MPH. Also, I'm deeply indebted to the generous information that the Alzheimer's Association provides in various sources, both in print and on the Web. But I went further. I joined the Alzheimer's Association and trained to become a volunteer presenter for their Speaker's Bureau to help inform others about the disease. In addition, I studied a number of books and online journal articles, attended university seminars that summarized current research, and read numerous news reports and magazine articles. A partial list of my resources is given in the Chapter Notes.

Alzheimer's disease has been likened to an epidemic, a "dementia time bomb," because it's spreading so rapidly throughout the United States. Eighty million baby boomers have become seniors at the rate of ten thousand a day since January 2011, and this rate will continue for nineteen years until 2030, when those sixty-five and older will make up 18 percent of the American population. Although age itself doesn't cause Alzheimer's, simply put, the longer one is alive, the more one is at risk. Already over 5.2 million Americans are estimated to be living with the disease, including 200,000 under the age of sixty-five, one in nine over the age of sixty-five, and one-half of those older than age eighty-five. Even these figures are probably too low, because, according to the Alzheimer's Association, AD may be under-diagnosed by about half. It's now ranked as the third leading cause of death in the United States, and it's the only disease among the top ten causes of death with no means so far to stop it, cure it, or even slow its progression *after* symptoms appear.

Current thinking is that preclinical Alzheimer's-like changes may begin as many as twenty or more years before symptoms appear, and typically there will be another twelve years between the onset of symptoms and diagnosis. This is a critical window for action, *before* early age-related memory losses become irreversible symptoms of disease. The time to prevent dementia is now, while brains are healthy and early prevention is still effective. Clearly there is no time to waste.

I'll share the steps I'm taking to fight against Alzheimer's disease. I hope you'll join me. Like my mother, I am "not going gently."

# CHRONOLOGY OF EVENTS IN MADELINE'S STORY

Born March 2, 1920
Married October 7, 1939

Chapter One:

| | |
|---|---|
| May 2002 | Parents become lost overnight in Nevada desert |
| January 2, 2005 | Death of Michael, her husband |
| January 6, 2005 | Madeline travels to Puerto Vallarta with author |
| May 2005 | Her first flight alone to visit author in CA |

Chapter Two:

| | |
|---|---|
| August 2005 | Madeline's second flight alone to visit author in CA |
| December 2005 | Her third flight alone to visit author in CA |
| March 2006 | Her last trip with author to Puerto Vallarta |
| May 2006 | She is moved to studio apartment in senior residence |

Chapter Three:

| | |
|---|---|
| May 2008 | Madeline's car trip with author and husband to CA |

# PART ONE

## MADELINE'S STORY

# CHAPTER ONE: LOST

## Warning Signs in Orientation and Recognition

On a Sunday night in May 2002, my parents, Madeline and Michael, went to their favorite restaurant for dinner and failed to return home. The disappearance of a couple in their mid-eighties would cause concern almost anywhere, but especially so in Nevada. There, new cities seemed to spring up overnight, like mirages on the edge of an otherwise featureless desert landscape. The town where my parents were living with my brother had recently been named the fastest growing city in the United States, and the joke was that residents who returned from a two-week vacation got lost because they couldn't recognize their own street. But missing elderly parents was clearly no joke.

Mom and Dad had lived in a small town in Pennsylvania almost their entire lives, a town with two-lane streets and few traffic lights. Now they were living in a megalopolis of uniformity. Every major intersection had the same look-alike commercial conglomerate, centered by a megastore with tentacles of smaller shops, restaurants, fast-food takeout, and offices. Even the first home my parents owned in Nevada was identical in its pastel stucco boxy shape to every other house in that development built for seniors. When my husband Ed went out for coffee early one morning the first time we visited there, he was glad he'd taken my father's car; coming back to their house, he'd had to click the garage door opener repeatedly as he drove down their street until he found the one door that opened. If my parents were confused and disoriented, they had good reason to be so in those surroundings. As their needs grew and their mental states weakened, my brother—also named Michael—a physician, moved them three more times in as many years until finally they were living with him in his large, new house.

When Michael came home from his meeting at the hospital the night they disappeared and discovered their absence, he immediately called his friend at the restaurant in the hope that Mom and Dad might still be there. "No," the friend said, "your parents left the restaurant a few hours ago." The restaurant was less than two miles from his house, and my brother had no idea where Mom and Dad could be.

Alarmed now, Michael called my two sisters and me in California to tell us our parents were missing. My husband Ed and I, who live in the San Francisco Bay area, happened to be in Southern California to attend a ceremony involving one of our granddaughters. We were staying with my sister Kate and her husband George, and the four of us were able to talk together with Michael on a speakerphone. My other sister, Patricia, who also lives in Southern California, wasn't speaking to Kate and me, so Michael, referring to himself as "neutral, like Switzerland," called her separately and relayed information back and forth. Between calls, all of us anxiously awaited more news. Meanwhile, as we pieced together what had probably happened and what could potentially happen to our parents, we became more and more frightened for them. We could only imagine how terrified they must have felt.

My mother would have been the one driving since my father had lost his sense of direction and stopped taking charge of everything a few years earlier, when he was in his early eighties. He was now eighty-four. If Mom, two years younger, had made a wrong turn when leaving the restaurant, only a few more wrong turns would have taken them out into the dark, dimensionless desert night, the city lights just a faint glow behind them in the distance. We were all panicked that they'd drive out of state and perhaps off a cliff someplace like the Grand Canyon. Hoover Dam was only a half hour away. Or perhaps they'd been kidnapped and robbed or were being held for ransom. Maybe someone had hijacked the car. Together we decided that Michael should report them missing to the Nevada police. As the long night wore on, we were even planning to hire a helicopter search team to look for them at daylight.

Mom and Dad drove around literally all night long, for at least ten hours. We have no idea how many miles they drove; surely they'd had to buy gas somewhere. By checking Dad's credit card activity, we learned that at some point after midnight they'd managed to find an open motel and check in. When we called the motel, the manager said that since they hadn't been able to locate their room, they'd gone back to the motel office so my dad could cancel the charge on his credit card. (We had a grim chuckle at this news: Dad may have been lost, but he wasn't about to lose money as well.) Surely, they must have been exhausted and needed to sleep; perhaps they slept in the car for a while. All we know is that early in the morning they eventually found a fast-food restaurant, where my mother entered and asked someone to call her son, the doctor, to come and get them.

I had reason to worry about them when they were flying, too, particularly since on two earlier occasions my parents had become lost inside the vast Las Vegas airport when they returned home from visiting me in California. My brother had been frantic each time, running and searching for them in that crowded airport until he finally caught sight of them, two frightened seniors no doubt holding on tightly to each other.

If we had ever questioned that Mom and Dad had crossed the line from the normal forgetfulness associated with age to mild cognitive impairment (MCI) or worse, we couldn't have had more dramatic evidence than their tendency to become lost. Later I learned that the ability to "map" might be lost before any memory changes occur. MCI doesn't necessarily lead to dementia, but it does require a professional cognitive evaluation. I was trusting that my brother Michael would take care of that.

In May 2005, my mother was traveling by herself for the first time since Dad had passed away five months earlier, in January. Eager to see her, I was prepared with an escort pass to meet her at the gate when her flight arrived at the San Jose airport. As I waited, I thought about her last trip, the day after Dad's funeral when Ed and I took her with us to our condo in Puerto Vallarta for two weeks so she wouldn't be home alone at Michael's house while he worked. One afternoon at the condo, I could hear Mom quietly sobbing as she lay on her bed. I was so sad to hear her crying. I gave her some time alone with her thoughts and emotions before I went into her room to talk to her about our grieving for my father. Imagine how amazed I was when she told me she didn't know Dad had died! I thought, *She must be in shock, denying the reality.* I didn't know what to do. Since she was apparently in distress, I felt I had to tell her the truth. But she wouldn't believe it until I reluctantly put the chip from my camera into my laptop and showed her some photos of the funeral. Then she quietly accepted the fact. Perhaps her earlier tears had been due to confusion because my dad wasn't with her and she didn't know where he was. These thoughts were in my mind as I anxiously awaited her arrival now in San Jose, not sure if my brother had stayed and watched until she boarded and the plane had taken off in Las Vegas.

At last I saw Mom coming, before she noticed me. "Thank goodness," I breathed, first in relief before thinking, "She's here, and she even remembered to carry her raincoat and purse off the plane." Yet happy as I was to see her, each time I was a little startled. Since she'd stopped coloring her hair and wearing much makeup a few years earlier, she was now a much paler, older version of her former self. But at eighty-five years of age, Madeline still walked with good posture and a light, although somewhat less confident, step. And she continued to have a trim figure and dress attractively, so the rest of her appearance was youthful in spite of the signs of age in her face and hair.

As soon as she saw me, she had a bright smile on her face—and a look of surprise. "You're here," she said, as we hugged each other. "How did you know to meet me here?" Then, before I could answer, she added, "When I woke up this morning, I decided I was going to visit my sister. You know, if you don't do these things when you think of them, they never happen at all."

Still thinking I was her sister, she continued, "Michael said, 'Mom, how do you think you'll visit your sister?' But I just told him, 'Watch and see; it'll work out.'"

I was shocked that she didn't recognize me yet afraid if I corrected her I might cause her to become upset or embarrassed and spoil her animated mood. She chatted happily during the thirty-minute drive to my house and asked me repeatedly when I, still meaning her sister, had moved so far away from the airport. I slowly and carefully interjected here and now reminders into the conversation so that by the time we arrived and she saw my husband Ed and the house we'd lived in for the past nine years, she seemed aware again of our identities and her surroundings.

When I called my brother later to let him know that Mom had arrived safely, I told Michael what she'd said at the airport. He wasn't surprised. "One day," he said, "she introduced me as, 'my brother, the butcher.'" Michael might be accustomed to Mom's confusion, but I was upset, especially since all but two of her seven siblings, including "the butcher" had passed away years ago. Which sister was I supposed to be? Who knew what year she thought it was or what time frame she was reliving? How long would it be before she was unable to recognize us as members of her family, even if the wrong ones? I went to bed that night quite shaken.

I used to think "change" was filled with optimism and hope. But at a certain point in life, the past begins to look a lot more attractive than the future. My mother had reached that point. A series of four moves in a little more than five years had taken her from being a wife and an independent homeowner with a house full of furnishings and accessories in Southern California—and an active life of driving, shopping, going to church, and enjoying visits from my two sisters and their husbands, who lived nearby—to a very secluded existence as a widow living with my divorced and childless only brother, in Nevada.

Mom had never wanted to give up her home in San Clemente and had resisted moving as long as she could. When my father became determined that they should move, Ed and I encouraged them to move near our home in Menlo Park where we could assist them if they needed anything. But my father thought the cost of living in the Bay Area was too high and insisted instead on relocating close to Michael, only partly for economic reasons.

Dad was certain Michael would take care of their physical needs for the rest of their lives, just as they had taken care of him by helping him financially through medical school and starting his own practice. Because of this conviction, Dad basically gave my brother total control over my parents' lives and finances once they moved to Nevada. Apparently my father had lost confidence in his own ability to make decisions, just as when he'd lost his sense of direction he turned all the driving over to my mother. What Dad thought was a simple and straightforward arrangement would turn out later to be very different from what he'd planned.

As Dad's health and Mom's memory deteriorated, they moved again and again, downsizing from a town home to a manufactured home, then to my brother's former house, and finally, in 2004, to one of the two master bedroom suites in my brother's beautiful new house. In retrospect, every one of these moves, although seemingly necessary and logical at the time, probably added to my parents' disorientation and perhaps also caused confusion and depression. Each time they moved, my mother lost more and more of her treasures. Worst for her was her loss of independence; she was angry for a long time after Michael had to take away her car keys and sell her car when she started becoming lost. In just five short years her life had been completely altered.

After Dad died, Mom wanted to continue living with Michael. She adored her youngest child, her only son, and imagined that since he was single, he'd also want to have company. But it was she who was alone with his dog Samson while Michael was at his office or at the hospital for so many hours each day. No doubt the solitude exacerbated her memory loss. But Mom said she wasn't ready "yet" to make any major changes in her living arrangements. She'd had a big enough adjustment to make, losing my father—her life partner and companion—after sixty-five years of marriage. For now the plan was for her to continue living with Michael but to periodically visit my two sisters and me in California.

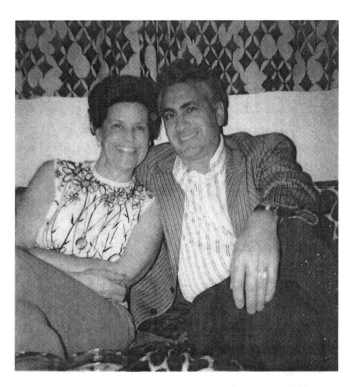

*Our parents, Madeline and Michael, Christmas Day 1972*

We'd always had wonderful times together when my parents visited my husband Ed and me after we moved to Northern California in 1988, especially during our many family holidays and parties over the years, but when Mother arrived for this visit, we'd recently sold our house and were getting ready to move to a much-smaller townhome. (Thinking of what Mom had endured, it was almost painful when she asked me, "Are you going to miss this house?") I wanted Mom to have a chance to enjoy the surroundings so familiar to her for one last visit before we began to pack our belongings.

My hope now was that the change of scenery plus the diversions from her everyday routines would be both pleasant and mentally stimulating for her. It wasn't long before I realized that keeping Mom stimulated for two weeks wasn't going to be as easy as it used to be when we still lived near each other in Southern California. I didn't have to be a psychologist to recognize that her memory had become worse than when she first was increasingly unable to retain parts of a conversation. At that time, I'd hoped some of her failure had to do with a lack of attention; I wasn't sure she was making the additional effort to put new information into memory that is often necessary as we age. But her problems had become more diffuse. Now if her difficulty with working memory (also called "short-term memory") was involving the prefrontal cortex, perhaps she was no longer *able* to pay attention.

Mother had lost interest in the activities that used to be her favorites, like going shopping. "I don't need anything more," she'd say. "I already have everything." This was probably true on a philosophical level, although I noticed that she could use a few little things, like a new black belt. Always a stylish dresser, she'd packed a navy-blue belt because she couldn't find the black one she needed, but the navy belt wasn't only a cheap plastic one, it showed excessive use. Still she didn't want to shop for a new belt, nor did she want to look for new shoes to replace the pair she said hurt her each time she wore them. A lifetime of thriftiness had hardened her against spending any money now, even when she could afford to shop. Mom still looked good, though, in spite of dressing herself a little too warmly for the season. Each day she wore nylon stockings, often with a wool skirt and a light knit top.

She couldn't remember that the month was May and frequently expressed surprise about the flowers and the sunshine in what she thought was winter. Her confusion about the season was remarkable, considering that she'd read the newspaper each morning and never notice the date or the day of the week. In fact, since she obviously hadn't absorbed anything from her reading, once she finished the news she'd start over again with the front page unless I stopped her by giving her a book to read in place of the paper. She never had been very interested in current events, but fortunately she still did like to read novels and could become so involved in a story that she'd skip watching her favorite daytime television show *Days of our Lives* or taking an infrequent afternoon nap in order to read a book. Reading, plus visiting my daughter Renée and her toddler boys, or having lunch out with me was enough to occupy her days now that she was more easily tired.

In the evenings, Ed and I often took her to a restaurant for dinner or to a movie theater. Sometimes I rented movies the three of us could watch together. One rental in particular was a beautiful love story called *The Notebook*, starring James Garner and Gena Rowlands. I didn't realize it at the time I chose this film, but the story involved the stars as an older married couple, she a victim of Alzheimer's disease in a nursing home and he a visitor who came faithfully to read to her every day, although she could neither remember nor recognize him. By the end of the movie, I was almost crying. Even my husband had tears in his eyes. But Mom sat on the sofa, dry-eyed and stoic. I asked her, "Don't you think the story was really sad?"

She said in a matter of fact way, "Well, I've seen this happen many times before. It's just a part of aging, and there's nothing you can do about it."

From time to time Mom would explain, "I used to have a very good memory, but I don't anymore." I asked her once if this was scary for her. She seemed puzzled by my question. To her, losing her memory was more of an annoyance than something to fear. Sometimes she seemed even to be amused by it.

When she referred to me as "her sister" on another occasion, I asked, "Mom, which sister am I supposed to be?"

"I don't know," she said with a grin. "I was hoping you'd tell me." If, in her mind, her children were young, then our middle-aged selves would naturally have seemed like we were her siblings, rather than her children.

I wasn't certain if Mom was aware that her memory loss had progressed and could become even worse. Or was she in denial? Her attitude was both brave and sad. I'd hoped for my mother to have the experience of independence and the freedom of being her own person after years of living with my father. But the time for her to make a new beginning seemed to have passed. Instead she did something that amazed me, but was almost as good, given her circumstances: she seemed to have completely obliterated any memory of past hurtful words and insults. When she spoke of Dad now, it was only of the good husband he'd become in his relatively becalmed later years and of how much she missed him. If Mom were going to lose some memories of her husband, at least she had the luck and the grace to remember only the better ones. (As I've learned, aging individuals tend to recall memories more positively.)

One sunny morning, hoping both to entertain her and to jog her other good memories a little, I brought out a large manila envelope filled with our family photos and a copy of her family's history, written by her oldest brother. We sat at the round glass table in the windowed alcove of my kitchen, the warm May sun shining in on us, and I showed Mom what I'd saved. At first she was delighted to see these pictures of her past. She exclaimed in awe over the photos of her long-dead parents. She was thrilled to see images of herself and my father when they were still very young. She struggled to identify her siblings and to remember which ones still survived. Then, all of a sudden, her joy and amazement at my having these photographs turned to anger. "These are my pictures," she said. "What are you doing with them?"

"You gave them to me. They were extras, and you said I could have them."

"But now you have them and I don't have any. These are of my family, and you took them from me."

We went back and forth like this a couple of times. I'd momentarily forgotten about her memory loss and was hoping that repetition would somehow help her to understand. Finally, I explained. I reminded her of the day, maybe six or seven years earlier, when I'd visited her and Dad while they were still living in San Clemente before they moved to Nevada. The three of us were sitting on their living room sofa together, going through a large box of photos I'd found in their garage. I was suggesting they might like to put some of these pictures into the still-empty photo albums I'd bought them some months earlier. I knew that this activity could be an interesting and valuable life review for seniors, and I thought that the two of them might enjoy doing it together. As far as I know, though, they never even started it. (My father, however, did write his memoirs at my urging, filling legal tablets in longhand for over a year. I typed his pages for him and gave him the only printed copy with the suggestion that he have copies made for my siblings. Alas, he never did, and when my computer crashed, I no longer had a copy either—or a back up, another irretrievable loss, this time due to my own negligence. Unfortunately, by then my parents had been living with my brother for a few years, and my father's only printed copy had also disappeared.)

"You should be glad that I still have these pictures," I finally told her. "Otherwise they would be lost, too." My words sounded harsher than I'd intended them to be, and I regretted them as soon as I'd said them. But the truth remained that along the way as my brother moved my parents from each location to another smaller one, more of their belongings disappeared each time. He took complete charge of their relocating, and, since my sisters and I lived out of state, he apparently didn't want to bother us and so didn't call on us to help. In fact, I usually heard about the latest move after the fact. Michael managed to somehow quietly discard everything he considered nonessential in order to fit the shrinking space available. Unfortunately, he included all mementos, saving nothing for my sisters and me except for the framed photos of our own families that we'd given Mom and Dad over the years. Perhaps other things had been sold, some given away, and some, as my mother strongly believed, were simply taken by unscrupulous movers and so-called helpers. (I'm not certain if this was the paranoia often associated with dementia or if it had some basis in truth. Both of my parents strongly suspected, and even gave me specific descriptions of, thefts by people who probably saw Mom and Dad as easy targets, too old and frail to notice their loss.)

The losses were especially hard on my mother, who'd always taken such good care of all her possessions. I remember in particular her set of stainless steel pans, evidently quite an expensive investment for her and my father when they'd purchased them sometime in the 1950s, probably with installment payments. She'd valued those pans so highly that she kept them polished like new for as long as she owned them. Now they, too, had disappeared, along with almost everything else she'd owned. She had a right to her anger, and who could blame her? Her memory, her possessions, her photos—all of this was lost from a woman who used to notice everything and who complained that a wooden spoon was missing when they moved from Pennsylvania to California in 1977. I did feel sorry for her; even more, my heart was breaking to think of where her journey was leading.

"Anyway," I added lamely, "aren't you happy that we still have these?"

She ignored my question. She'd gone back to shuffling through the photos, laying them out on the table in front of her like playing cards. My original separation of her birth family from ours into two distinct groups of pictures was now lost, making it harder for her to recognize people. She had to ask me over and over again to identify even those near and dear to her. At times she was unable to recognize my two younger sisters as children or even as teens. Apparently my brother and I stood out—he was the only male child, and I was her first born, making me the only one whose name she'd written on the back of my baby photos. (No wonder she'd always told me to write names and dates on the backs of pictures to remember who was in the photo, but even so, I couldn't imagine ever being unable to recognize family members.) In a sudden gesture of sharing, she decided to return my early pictures to me now. Perhaps she understood that the real loss was her memory and without it, the pictures really meant nothing.

As I watched her I began to realize that as her memory faded, so did the portion of those lives to which only she held the final link. So much of what we'd shared was already gone; questions I might like to ask about my early childhood would remain forever unanswered. It was as though the part of a life that no one remembers no longer exists. And what about her parents and siblings who'd passed away? If we live on in others' memories, then is their loss of memory our final obliteration?

I couldn't help but wonder about my own future. How long until I, like my mother, might lose my memory? Twenty years or less? I was already concerned whenever I couldn't recall words, especially names, since memory can begin to decline around the age of forty-five. During menopause when hot flashes at night kept me awake, I'd experienced the sensation of "brain fog," suddenly going blank during the day, a most disturbing sensation if it were to happen while I was teaching a college class. My symptoms stopped suddenly when my doctor prescribed hormone replacement therapy. Within a day of taking the pills I felt like I had my mind back again. Yet my experience was just a dress rehearsal compared to what my mother had already endured.

Loss of names leads to loss of identity, first that of others, then of one's own. Without memories to define us, who are we to ourselves and to our loved ones? How long until my own life wouldn't only be over, but also faded from others' memories? Even worse would be a living death—consciousness without memory. That last thought was a cold knife of fear in my core, for both my mother and myself.

After some time, distressed by these thoughts, I left her with the pictures in the kitchen and went into the room we called our library. I needed a distraction and wanted to sort through the contents of some cabinets in preparation for packing later. Soon I had a stack on the coffee table of old travel folders and maps to be thrown away; I was glad that at least this much was ready for the trash before we took the cans out to the curb for pick up the following morning.

Not until lying in bed that night did I realize I hadn't seen the manila envelope with the family photos since our morning in the kitchen. Worried, I got out of bed and went downstairs to look for it, but I couldn't find it anywhere. I finally went back to bed, and then the thought occurred to me—what if the envelope had somehow become mixed in with the trash from the library and had been thrown away? I made a mental note to wake before the trash was collected, and dawn found me outside in my bathrobe, searching through all those papers that fortunately were on top of the garbage. No manila envelope, no pictures, no family history appeared, so I reasoned that probably Mom had taken them to her room.

Later, after she came downstairs and had had her breakfast and morning pills, I mentioned the envelope to Mom and asked her if she had put it in her suitcase. She didn't remember, so we went up to her room and looked—under the bed, under the mattress, in the bureau drawers, in her bathroom. My mother's gift for hiding was legendary. Sometimes we'd receive a Christmas gift in the middle of summer when, as she'd say, "I finally ran across where I hid this." Now either the experience of losing things or maybe her growing dementia had driven her to hide everything she could against possible intruders who she feared might come and steal from her.

She had hidden their diamond rings--both hers and my father's--somewhere in my brother's house but then forgot where, and years later they still haven't been found. In spite of our careful searching, however, we failed to find the envelope of photos, and I felt sick, thinking that it must have been in the trash after all, and decades of memories were gone forever.

I fretted about this loss of the family photos and history for days. Mom, however, didn't appear to be disturbed. In fact, after our search, she seemed to have forgotten all about them, as if they, too, had been sucked into some black hole in the brain where memories disappear.

Soon the time came for Mom to leave us and return to Michael's house. This was always a sad and difficult time for her and for me, but especially so since she was so vulnerable now. We hated to part; I worried about her security and comfort, and she would lose my constant companionship. Even a short, one-hour flight could stress and disorient her, causing her to ask me over and over again the same questions about the time and details of her trip. Again at the airport I obtained an escort pass so I could wait with her at the gate. When it was time for her to board, she had tears in her eyes as she hugged me tight. So did I.

But there was work to do at home. Ed and I had to pack as much as we could before the movers came. We started upstairs with the easy rooms—the guest bedrooms and baths, the hall closet. We gave boxes of books to the town library, clothes to one charity, household items and excess furniture to another charity or to some of the five adult children in our blended family. Next we worked on our office, and the task became much more difficult. Ed had to part with decades of business and financial records. At least those were completely impersonal, and he wasn't bothered giving them up as long as the documents were shredded. But the records I had to throw away—old lecture notes and papers from almost thirty years of college teaching—felt very personal to me, especially since my primary field of developmental psychology bore such a close parallel to my real life. Letting go was a painful process. Sometimes I still think about and search in vain for some of those materials.

I felt like chunks out of our past were being jettisoned.

As I worked on the packing, I thought about my mother's question, "Will you miss this house?" The answer was finally no, I wouldn't miss the house. Really, the house was just a shell that held the special events and the living that we'd done in it. What I'd miss were all the fun and activities we'd enjoyed during these past nine years. Logically, this move made so much sense, although emotionally I *did* feel a sense of loss—not of the material aspects, but of the years gone by, the period of life that was over, the vitality and energy we'd expended. All of the good times seemed to be behind us. Our children and grandchildren were the key actors in the family now, and we had become the observers—off stage, but thankfully still in the audience.

To my thinking, the big decisions in life had already been made. They were good ones, for the most part, having brought us to this point. But no more major crossroads lay ahead. We already knew whom we'd marry, how many children we'd have, what our careers would be, where we'd live. One by one, our choices had been made, paths taken, direction set. Now the future held time for only small choices.

When had "change" become synonymous with "loss"? But, in truth, was this not what all the holding on—to pictures, to possessions—was about? Were we not all afraid, consciously or unconsciously, of the ultimate letting go? We were making this move just two years after Ed had been diagnosed with third-stage lung cancer and our lives had changed dramatically. Ed sold our businesses, and I stopped teaching classes at Santa Clara University. Our days were centered on making the raw food smoothies and other lifestyle changes that had brought him back to health. Now, downsizing itself seemed to move us one step closer to the advent of old age. Nor did it help to know that we were buying the town house from a couple who, like so many others in that town-house association, were selling in order to move into a retirement hotel with assisted living options. For them, only a final act remained to answer the last questions of life.

For my father, those questions had been answered in a rehabilitation center four months after he fell one night in his bathroom and broke his hip. My mother visited Dad every day in the rehabilitation center, staying with him, helping to feed him lunch, chatting with the nurses, and leaving when the driver my brother had hired came to pick her up. Because of his knee pain, Dad was never able to do the therapy exercises my brother said he had to complete before coming home. Dad passed away in the rehabilitation center on January 2, 2005, just nineteen days after his eighty-seventh birthday.

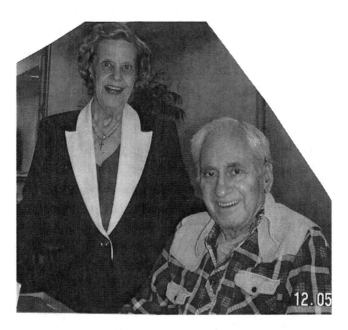

These grim thoughts of loss and death weren't part of my usual nature. I knew that once I was settled into our new home I'd forget such sadness and instead look ahead with more optimism. But in the back of my mind I couldn't help but again be reminded that in twenty years I might be very much like my mother and my father. Would I have their same stoicism and be able to accept, as Mom had said, "There's nothing you can do about it," or would I fight against loss and age and death until the end?

Finally, the day arrived when the packers came to finish the work Ed and I had started. We had stayed on the perimeter, packing the easy things; the Irish workers from the moving company were fanning out and attacking the very heart of the house. I walked from room to room to see each setting, each room's unique arrangement and decor one last time before its contents would disappear into boxes and its furniture dispersed.

My favorite room was our so-called library, a sort of family/media room. This was our place for informal gatherings—watching football games and TV shows, opening Christmas gifts, encouraging babies as they took their first steps. Of the five children in our family, the last two to be married were wed when Ed and I lived in this house, and we held all the accompanying engagement parties and showers here. Our seven youngest grandchildren (of our total twelve grandchildren) were born while we lived here (and as toddlers learned to open the special cabinet in the kitchen where I kept a basket of toys for them). This was the only "Mimi and Papa's house" they'd ever known.

We called this room a library because two opposing walls were lined with mahogany bookshelves and cabinets. Never again would I have a room that could hold so much. But then, never again would I have so much to hold. Here were all of my carefully organized photo albums, more than forty years of our lives arranged in chronological order, linking fragmented episodes into a chain of continuity. Those pictures reminded me of what we were like at our happiest moments and helped me to actually relive the events in my mind. They held the moments of time that will never come again, touchstone memories, the only things I could really keep—but for how long? I could certainly understand Mom's reaction to her pictures. If I could have put each photo under lock and key instead of merely affixing it to a page, I would have.

Standing there in the library, reflecting, I lost my composure. Ian, one of the Irish movers, noticed the tears in my eyes and gallantly said, "Having a bit of the allergies today, are we?" I nodded and retreated quickly, upstairs to my bedroom, to wait until Ian was finished with the very last thing left to do, disconnecting the stereo components and television in the library.

When I came back downstairs after the packers had left, the house I saw was no longer mine. It was just a place filled with shrink-wrapped furniture and lots of boxes. Propped in front of one box on the piano bench was a manila envelope. I didn't have to look to know that it contained Mom's pictures and history. Ian had found it where she'd hidden it, evidently behind the stereo equipment. Mom hadn't taken any more chances. She'd tried her best and done the only thing she knew to do in order to hold on to the last images of her past. In the end, memory had failed her after all.

It wasn't until a few months later, after we were settled into our new home (happily so, I might add), that I emptied the contents of the manila envelope onto my desk. My intention was to make copies of my mother's favorite photos and give them to her in a small album held together by ribbon; fortunately, enough good photos remained for me to create this keepsake and present it to her.

But to my surprise, one of the pictures she liked the best, a photo of her with my father when they were young, wasn't even in the envelope with the others. She'd had enough memory left to recognize and hide the one that meant the most to her. Eventually, I found it—tucked into a book she'd been reading when she visited us. My mother may have been losing her memory, but she'd kept her cunning ability to hide things—if only she could have remembered where.

Would we be able to save her from any more losses?

# CHAPTER TWO: LONELY

## Need for Social Interaction and Emotional Support

Mother traveled alone by plane twice more in 2005 to visit Ed and me in California. In late August, we watched the Katrina disaster together as it unfolded on television. Sometimes Mom and I would bring a picnic lunch to a nearby park and walk around the lovely lagoon there. In December, we prepared for the coming holidays, selecting and decorating a Christmas tree for what would be our last time doing this together. The photo shows her pleasure just after she and I had successfully completed a large puzzle of colorful flowers.

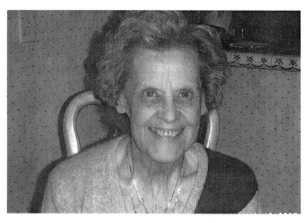

During these two visits, Mom continued to show some confusion and problems with memory; she often repeated conversations. But she was generally happy and needed little supervision. If only I had known what was going to happen. If only I could have kept her like that.

Instead, five months after Christmas, my sister Kate and I were stunned to receive surprising news. Mother had been moved yet again, this time from Michael's home into a rather large residential-care home for seniors in Nevada.

Kate and I weren't aware that our sister Patricia (who, like Kate, still lives in Southern California) had taken such a major role in decision making with our brother. But Patricia had helped Michael find a care home, furnish the small studio apartment they had selected within it, and move Mother there, all without our knowledge. Two years later we heard their justification: it wasn't good for Mother to be alone all day while Michael worked. We could all agree to that reason. But this wasn't the way it was supposed to be.

Years ago my father had purchased a home health-care policy so that neither he nor my mother would ever have to be placed into a care home for seniors. With this insurance, he reasoned, they could live out their lives among family, specifically living with Michael in his home as had long been planned. Health-care workers could be hired to come in and assist either or both parents when necessary. Instead, Dad's wishes had been ignored.

Michael didn't want "strangers," as he called them, coming to his house while he was at work, so he and Patricia listed Mother's home address at the senior residence center. Instead of providing in-home, personal, or companion care, "so that elderly adults can continue to live independently in their own homes throughout America," as advertised, the "visiting angel" Patricia hired would visit Mom in her new studio apartment at the residential-care home each weekday for a few hours of companionship.

Now instead of being with her family, Mom was going to live among strangers and have a part-time companion who had no knowledge of her as a person or of her past. Even her most basic identity, her name, would be left behind. From now on, instead of having been called "Lee" all her life by those close to her, my mother would be known as "Madeline."

To say my mother liked or approved of this arrangement would be a complete denial of the truth. Many times in the past she'd told me that she would never want to live among other old people; she wanted to stay close to young people with their energy and zest for life. So she resisted. Michael reported that he had to stop taking her to his home for visits. Mom would be so angry and belligerent when it was time to take her back to her apartment at the senior residence that she'd become physically aggressive, fighting and struggling to remain in his house where she'd lived for a few years. One time, she actually hid under her former bed, Michael told me, and he'd had to physically drag her out and put her in his car.

No, Mom would not go gently.

My mother had devoted her life to my father and to us, her four children. Born in 1920, she was the second youngest in a family of two sons and six daughters. She was also the darling of a childless aunt and uncle who brought Lee to live with them in Cleveland when she was in junior high school. The following year when she wanted to return home to western Pennsylvania, she was unable to transfer her grades and records between schools in different states. Unwilling to repeat a grade, she dropped out of school after the eighth grade. She stayed at home with her parents and younger sisters until she was old enough to get a job. Then, for a few years she worked at a five-and-dime store. One summer night she met my father at a romantic lakeside casino dance. She married him a year later, when she was nineteen, and quit the only paying job she ever had.

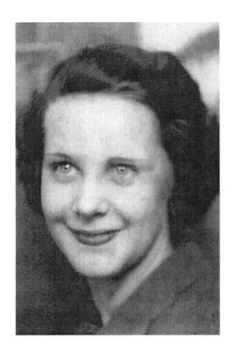
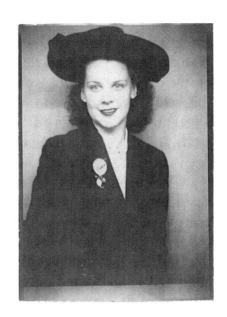

I was born a year after their wedding. The next child was Patricia, then Kate, each of us five years apart in age. Michael, the long-awaited male child, was born when I was seventeen and literally graduating from high school. In fact, my mother was still in the hospital with Michael the night of my graduation and missed the big party for me she'd so gallantly prepared in advance. Following my graduation, I had a summer job in a department store and was desperately praying to find a scholarship in order to leave home and attend college in the fall. Patricia, therefore, became the second mother to Michael, just as I'd been to Kate. Little did we know that these early bonds would foretell an alignment of us siblings in our later adult years that affected our abilities—or desire—to communicate with one other.

Over the years we became separated even more by both physical distance and temperament. After I went away to college (a scholarship did arrive) I never really lived at home any more. I started my own family soon after my graduation from Ohio University, and since my firstborn, Mark, is only four years younger than my brother Michael, I've always felt more like an aunt to my brother. Patricia and I became very close friends when we were the first two in our family who moved to California. She followed me by a year, in 1967; the others didn't leave Pennsylvania for another ten years. But due to misunderstandings with each of us thirty years later, Patricia stopped all contacts with Kate and me and refused my subsequent attempts for reconciliation. I missed her friendship, her sense of humor, and all the good times we'd had together, but as years went by and she wasn't to be appeased, I finally had to accept the estrangement and let her go. Kate had an unenviable position in the family, growing up between Patricia and Michael, the youngest child and long-awaited only son, on whom my parents doted. In short, we weren't a good group to cooperate with one another in taking care of our mother.

The ideal would have been if I, or one of my siblings, could have taken Mother into one of our homes and cared for her, but for various reasons, no one had the right space or could provide the full-time responsibility. Ed and I had sold our big house while both of my parents were still living with Michael; we'd assumed they'd stay with him as my parents had planned, and now our small guest bedroom was filled with built-ins—bookshelves, a television, and a wall bed. The way we'd reconfigured it, our home no longer included a proper guest-room suite for Mom's permanent residence. Kate's house had a long flight of stairs to the guest-room suite, Michael worked, and Patricia had her own reasons. Ed and I thought we could keep Mom comfortable with us for three months at a time, but our idea of having Mom divide her year among us on a quarterly basis was considered by my other three siblings to be too confusing for her. She deserved so much more than we were ready to provide.

Residential care was not an easy solution. To me, it was heart wrenching; not to live up to our obligation and duty seemed so selfish and ungrateful of us. I had many feelings of grief and guilt, and I imagine my siblings felt the same way. Even more, I felt shame when I learned that seven out of ten patients with Alzheimer's disease live at home. Out of Mother's four children, not one of us was willing and able to give her the care she'd given us.

And so our Mother was sent away from her family. To explain what this abrupt change of living must have meant to her, let me go back and describe our experience with her in March 2006, just past her eighty-sixth birthday and two months prior to her placement in the senior residence. Ed and I had brought Mother with us again for another two weeks' vacation in Puerto Vallarta. She and my father had visited there with us many times before, so on this visit she was delighted to see again the friends she'd made in previous years. She enjoyed going to restaurants and the botanical gardens, and just generally relaxing, sitting on the balcony in the sun, looking out at the glistening bay and the huge pelicans flying in their V formation on the way to roost in the late afternoons, so close we could almost reach out and touch them. We watched television shows together and a movie she'd liked very much, *Forrest Gump*. None of us would have dreamed that this was to be her last trip to Mexico.

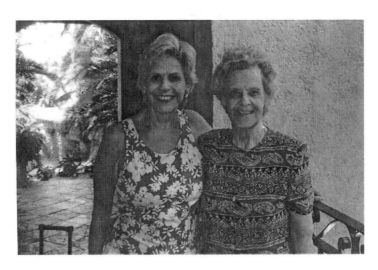

Then, only two months after our return from Puerto Vallarta where she and I had been constant companions, Mom was moved into the senior residence. Almost all of my subsequent visits with her for the next two years were in her studio apartment there.

The physical aspects of the apartment were actually quite pleasing and well located for my mother—on the first floor, around the corner from the spacious lobby/sitting area, almost directly across from the reception desk outside of the dining room; she wouldn't get lost. She enjoyed being able to sit and watch the activity in the lobby as people came and went, and every day she could go outside and take her walks around the large building.

Inside, Patricia and Michael had done a nice job of furnishing the apartment with Mom's sofa, dining table and chairs, television, coffee table, and accessories in the living area; on the bedroom side of the half wall were her queen-size bed, a large dresser, and nightstands. The bedroom window looked out on the circular driveway at the front of the building. The bathroom was fairly large, and there was a kitchenette with a microwave and a small refrigerator in one corner of the living area.

At least once every three months, I'd fly to Las Vegas, rent a car, and stay with Mom usually two days and a night (both of us sleeping together in her bed as it gave me the opportunity to spend as much time as possible with her). While there, I tried to give her the stimulation and activities of her previous life, and we had a great time together. I'd take her out shopping, sightseeing, to a hairdresser or a movie, and always to restaurants for lunch and dinner—my compromise and efforts since I was now one of the 15 percent of family or friends who are long-distance caregivers, living more than an hour away.

These visits gave me the chance to observe Mom in her own surroundings. Always a rather shy and private person, my mother didn't make friends easily. Although she was very likeable and had a few close friends when she was younger, after she moved to California in 1977 her friends were mainly her family, and she depended on us for most of her social activities. Ed and I had been particularly close to my parents, both socially and physically, when we lived in Laguna Beach and they lived nearby in San Clemente. We often took trips with Mom and Dad, not only to Puerto Vallarta, but also once or twice to Arizona. For my father's eightieth birthday, my parents, Kate and George (Kate's husband), Michael, Ed and I went on a riverboat cruise, visiting Civil War battlefields throughout the South from Nashville to Memphis. Ed and I celebrated every holiday and birthday together with Mom and Dad and the rest of our extended family. My parents even watched our children for us when Ed and I went away for a weekend. Unfortunately, after we moved to the Bay Area in 1988, we didn't see them as often, although they often came north to visit us, just as we traveled south to see them.

In contrast, at the senior residence, Mom lived in a virtual solitary confinement. She didn't participate in any of the activities such as field trips or craft classes or simple games like bingo (which she hated; the only games she used to like were card games such as Hearts that she played with my younger daughter, Renée). She didn't have a single close acquaintance or friend at the care home except her visiting angel who came for about an hour each weekday. Her meal companions were a difficult pair: Dorothy was deaf, and Joanne, who was terminally ill, smiled sadly but didn't speak. The fourth person at their table was quite lively and gregarious, but she soon had asked to be moved to another table, and no one else had ever taken, or probably had ever wanted to take, her place. Mom had learned to mask her confusion with silence as often as possible. Needless to say, there was never any conversation during dinner, the one time of day Mother mingled with others, and to my knowledge, none of us had ever requested moving her to another table.

After one of my early visits, on October 2, 2006, I wrote "Living in a Timeless Present":

> Today would have been my mother's sixty-
> seventh wedding anniversary, yet my mother doesn't

know it. Far from keeping a mental record of dates to celebrate, she usually doesn't know the day of the week—or even the season, for that matter.

Since my father passed away and she was moved into a senior care residence, all the usual markers of time passing in the outside world are missing to her, and now every day is the same.

She's with other people who have families different from hers. These families celebrate different anniversaries and birthdays of people she has never met and never will. Nor will her new companions ever know my mother's family—her children, her five grandchildren, her nine great-grandchildren. For all of those living in this place, these celebrations are held outside and no longer include them.

Each one of these women (for they are mainly women) lives in a solitary circle, her past contained and sealed, not touching the present, the future, or one another.

How could she have known it's her anniversary today? How would you celebrate if no one were there to celebrate with you?

So much of what we know about ourselves we learn by interacting with others. How we respond, how they in turn relate to us, are all part of discovering what makes us unique individuals. Identity is forged and maintained by social interactions. In this sense, then, isolation is a form of torture that can lead to losing the sense of self.

Certainly the staff didn't provide much social stimulation. During the times when I spent the night there with Mom, an aide would unlock her door and enter the room shortly after seven each morning, wake Mom, check to make sure her limbs were all working, give her some pills, and then leave after ten or fifteen minutes. My mother was becoming a little careless about her personal hygiene, but the aide didn't always stay to help make sure she showered and changed her clothes regularly.

I had never seen the contract with the residence center so I had no idea what services to expect from them until I found a list of their duties in one of Mom's dresser drawers. The duties covered considerably more than what they were doing. For example, a podiatrist was supposed to take care of Mom's feet and cut her toenails monthly. Yet I had to cut her toenails once because they were bothering her. No wonder. Their length reminded me of pictures of Howard Hughes's fingernails. Then I discovered something sharp under one of her toes. She had hammertoes, and the long nail of one was jabbing into the toe below it. Walking must have been extremely painful.

During her two years in the senior residence, I realized that her memory was becoming noticeably worse. Quite likely it would have continued to slowly deteriorate in that period wherever she lived, but I believe her memory loss was exacerbated because of her lack of social stimulation and the loss of extended contact with her family. Studies have shown that one of the best things we can do for our brains is to maintain social connections and engagements with family and friends as long as possible. Experts agree that when seniors become more isolated, issues of loneliness and depression can affect their memory and cognitive function.

In a six-year University of California San Francisco (UCSF) study of 1,604 older adults,[3] those who were lonely were more likely to develop difficulties performing activities of daily living like dressing and bathing themselves and had an increased risk of death. A similar study in Holland linked loneliness to cognitive decline and a greater likelihood of developing dementia. In both studies, more important than the number of people surrounding the individual was the sense of having strong emotional connections and the perception of a meaningful relationship.

One time I gave Mother some very informal cognitive questions. Previously she had lost an accurate sense of time (date, season, year, month). Now she'd also become confused with her immediate location as her spatial memory declined, probably indicating more loss of parietal lobe function. She didn't know where she lived, not even the state. She couldn't find her way around her building except to go to the dining room, fortunately almost directly across the hall from her room. In fact, she didn't seem to know where she was at any given moment, but she did know that she wasn't at home with her family. Most shocking, she could no longer recognize Dad in the large photo of him on her wall; she guessed he was her father. Was this a problem with her memory or with her vision? When I asked her who was president, she said, "Nixon."

Since she had regressed in those two years of semi-solitude, she'd require additional help now wherever she lived. She no longer turned on her television set or made calls on her phone (thankfully she could still answer my calls, and we had evening chats several times a week). She stopped reading books and newspapers. She quit washing her own hair, but Michael had arranged and paid for her to periodically go to the hair salon at the end of her hall.

In fact, she was exhibiting many of the ten warning signs quoted from the Alzheimer's Association list as harbingers of the disease:

- Memory loss that disrupts daily life: forgetting dates or events, asking for the same information over and over, relying on memory aids
  - Normal aging: Temporarily forgetting names or appointments
- Challenges in planning or in solving problems: Changes in ability to work with numbers, follow a recipe, track bills
  - Normal aging: Occasional mistakes when balancing a checkbook
- Difficulty in completing familiar tasks: Trouble driving somewhere familiar, managing a budget, remembering rules of a game
  - Normal aging: Occasionally needing help with settings such as TV recordings

- Confusion with time or place: Losing track of dates or seasons, forgetting where they are or how they got there
  - Normal aging: Getting confused temporarily about the day or the week
- Trouble understanding visual images or spatial relationships: Difficulty reading, judging distance, determining color
  - Normal aging: Vision changes from cataracts
- New problems with words in speaking and in writing: Trouble following or joining a conversation, repeating oneself
  - Normal aging: Sometimes having trouble finding the right word
- Misplacing things and losing the ability to retrace steps: Putting things in unusual places, accusing others of stealing
  - Normal aging: Occasionally misplacing things and retracing steps to find them
- Decreased or poor judgment: Bad moves with money, less attention to grooming
  - Normal aging: Making a bad decision once in a while
- Withdrawal from work or social activities
  - Normal aging: Sometimes feeling weary of work, family, and social obligations
- Changes in mood or personality: Becoming confused, suspicious, depressed, fearful, or anxious.
  - Normal aging: Becoming irritable when a specific routine is disrupted

On the other hand, she was still continent, and she was able to shower and dress herself. She also could certainly eat on her own, walk, and climb stairs. All of these are important abilities because they show she was still able to independently perform the six basic activities of daily living (ADL) used to measure level of functioning: eating, bathing, dressing, walking, toileting, and continence.

She would not have been able, however, to manage the more instrumental activities of daily living (IADL) such as shopping, preparing food, doing laundry, driving or using other transit, and managing finances. Although these abilities are essential for independent living, their loss doesn't necessarily mean it's time for residential care. More than one geriatrician has pointed out what Dr. Cathy Alessi says, "A lot of older people with impairment in these areas can remain relatively independent in the community if they can get the right kind of help...Your parent is still an independent person. Even a person with early or moderate dementia still has needs and wants and opinions, and they need to be respected."[4]

Mother's life was spent alone in her small apartment or in the lobby outside of the dining room, except for mealtimes and visits from one of us or from her visiting angel. Michael and his new wife Agnes dropped by to see her at least every week (they were married a few months after Mom entered the senior residence). Agnes, a recent immigrant, was very kind to my mother and called her "Mommy."

Agnes and my brother took treats for Mom to keep in her refrigerator or cupboard, but then Mom would forget to eat them. She began to wrap items in tissues and hide them in her increasingly disorganized dresser drawers, indicating the suspicion of others that often goes with worsening dementia but—along with becoming reclusive—may also be a sign of depression, a common affliction among the elderly that is often treatable and is sometimes mistaken for AD. Kaiser Permanente, in a long-term study of over thirteen thousand adults,[5] estimated that late-life depression might double the risk of Alzheimer's dementia; both depression and dementia cause damage or shrinkage to the hippocampus, the part of the brain so important for memory formation.

Still, she was registered at the senior residence as "independent" (because she had the outside help of a visiting angel) and wasn't in their "assisted living" program (which would have suggested more care and supervision from the staff). This distinction would become very important, as we were to discover later.

# CHAPTER THREE: LACKING

## Nutrition, the Brain, and Memory Changes

From the time Mother had moved into the senior residence two years earlier, she had not traveled outside of the immediate area of where she lived. In order for her to travel alone by plane to visit us, either my brother Michael or his wife Agnes would have had to take her to the airport and wait with her until the flight left, then be at the gate again when it was time for her return. Since that would be quite an inconvenience in their work schedules, I always visited her in her studio apartment where she lived, but my trips there were usually for only two or three days at a time.

To give Mother a longer visit, Ed and I decided to bring her home with us for a vacation. On April 26, 2008, we drove to Mother's residence center and packed her clothes, pills, and whatever else she might need for her stay, and the following day the three of us left for our home in California. I was looking forward to spending extended time with her again, but the extra days together would sadly reveal the many ways in which my mother's care had been lacking in fulfilling her needs.

We had intended to break the nine-hour drive by stopping somewhere to spend the night, but Mom was ready to continue on and complete the trip in one day. She seemed quite interested in the passing scenery and made appreciative comments about the changing views, although most of the time she was silent. When she did speak, she repeated conversations over and over again since she couldn't remember what had just been said. As usual, when in the car she'd exclaim periodically, "Look at all of these cars! Where do they all come from?" I think part of her pleasant demeanor was due to the many social skills she still had, skills that my brother said helped to conceal the extent of her memory loss. We couldn't tell whether this was an adventure for her or a confusing change of environment. In either case, she seemed happy.

Mother adjusted to her new surroundings in our home very well. Her only physical complaint, other than saying her right knee hurt (arthritis, whenever she got into or out of the car), was feeling dizzy and faint quite often. Possibly these symptoms were due to hypothyroidism, medications, or blood pressure; she'd had similar symptoms at times over the years. I checked with Michael to find out what prescription medications she was taking and then looked up their side effects:

- Cerefolin (for generic nutritional deficiencies associated with cognitive impairment in the elderly) can cause drowsiness, mild diarrhea, and body swelling.
- Benicar (for high blood pressure) can commonly cause dizziness, especially in the elderly, as well as feeling faint or nauseous.
- Aricept (for confusion related to dementia and Alzheimer's disease) can commonly cause nausea and diarrhea.
- Synthroid (a hypothyroid medication) can cause headaches and nervousness.

While Benicar would seem to have been the most likely cause of her feeling faint and dizzy, the thyroid pill seemed to be the one associated with her periods of feeling worse. I stopped giving it to her for a few days because I knew that my own thyroid supplement also could make me feel a bit queasy at times, and I wrote to

Michael to ask his opinion. I had not asked Michael what vitamins and supplements Mother was taking, but I suspected none, since I hadn't found any among her pills.

I believe that in addition to lacking adequate social stimulation and companionship in the assisted living residence, Mother was also lacking key elements in her diet and supplements. But as I was now learning, the time to slow her furthering dementia by giving her additional nutrients had sadly passed. Even the medication Aricept (donepezil) that Michael had prescribed was fast losing its effectiveness. In their material, the Alzheimer's Association states that cholinesterase inhibitors like Aricept, given to prevent the breakdown of the important memory transmitter acetylcholine, only delay symptoms for a limited time, an average of six to twelve months for about 50 percent of users.

Past efforts to treat patients with various drugs have not worked, it's now widely believed, primarily because they've been given too late. Alzheimer's doesn't suddenly begin in one's sixties or seventies. With the progress made in brain imaging and other biomarkers, Dr. Peter V. Rabins says, "Alzheimer's disease can be detected in a person's cerebrospinal fluid 10 to 25 years before people even have symptoms; most experts now agree that changes in certain biomarkers may precede Alzheimer's symptoms by as many as 30 years!"[6] By the time a person is diagnosed with even mild Alzheimer's-related dementia—with impaired short-term memory and some difficulty in daily functioning—he or she has already lost a significant amount of the neurons responsible for healthy memory and reasoning.

I had to finally accept that, for my mother, the time for prevention had passed.

Unfortunately, in spite of the advances in early detection, medications and therapies have lagged far behind. To date, AD is not treatable. No drugs to prevent, or even to slow, the progression of dementia exist, although new drugs are being tested in clinical trials. No one is claiming yet to cure dementia, especially its most common form—Alzheimer's disease—but hope does remain that in the future, the risk of AD may be lowered with medication and lifestyle changes, just as the risks of stroke and heart attack have been. Until then, in the absence of effective medication, how do we prevent dementia before its symptoms occur?

✳✳✳

A growing but still controversial number of studies indicate a correlation exists between taking certain nutritional supplements and delaying the onset of cognitive decline,[7] particularly for age-associated memory impairment. If I was already too late to help my mother, then perhaps the time had come for me to think about protecting my own cognitive health. These recommendations don't have the same FDA approval required for prescription drugs, however, and have not been proven in randomized trials. But given the hope of preventing or at least delaying possible future memory loss, I see no harm in trying to include at least some of the most frequently suggested key dietary supplements in my own daily regimen:

- B vitamins—especially $B_6$, $B_{12}$, and folic acid—that studies show help control high levels of the amino acid homocysteine associated with cognitive decline and Alzheimer's
- Vitamin $D_3$, since recent studies have shown a correlation between low levels of Vitamin $D_3$ and dementia; Vitamin $D_3$ has been found to be even more beneficial than Vitamin C, CoQ10, Acetyl L-Carnitine, and beta carotene (precursor of Vitamin A). (Vitamin E, once recommended, is now considered problematic, especially in high doses.)
- Glutathione, the "master antioxidant," to fight free radicals and slow vascular changes
- Essential fatty acids, especially omega-3, for their anti-inflammatory and antioxidant affects
- Alpha-lipoic acid, another beneficial antioxidant

Even better than taking pills is eating a Mediterranean diet high in fruits, vegetables, and whole grains and low in saturated fats, meats, dairy products and sugar. Several epidemiological reviews have reported that those who follow the Mediterranean diet lower their risk of Alzheimer's disease by 40 percent.[8] Especially important are foods rated high in antioxidants and rich in flavonoids, like blueberries and strawberries (a controlled six-year study of sixteen thousand women over the age of seventy showed two servings a week could delay cognitive decline by up to two and a half years),[9] and other so-called brain foods, including spices like dried oregano, ground cinnamon, and turmeric. Turmeric, the spice that turns curry yellow, with its active ingredient curcumin, is generally credited with the much lower incidence in India of Alzheimer's disease. And mice that were fed curcumin in a UCLA study years ago had half as many of the amyloid plaques of Alzheimer's disease as the control group.[10] The Alzheimer's Association website lists other protective foods for a healthy brain:

- Vegetables—kale, spinach, Brussels sprouts, broccoli, beets, red bell pepper, onion, corn, and eggplant
- Fruits—prunes, raisins, berries (blue, black, raspberries and strawberries), plums, oranges, red grapes, and cherries
- Fish—salmon, halibut, mackerel, trout, and tuna
- Nuts—almonds, pecans, and walnuts

What you eat and how much you eat are very important, therefore, for your brain as well as for your overall health. We have already noted the importance of social interactions and emotional support in my mother's case. Now we can add diet and supplements as a third critical factor for delaying memory loss and cognitive decline.

We cannot deny, however, that some memory changes do occur naturally. I have to admit that I still worry at times about my memory, in spite of my own healthy diet and supplements, a mentally stimulating and physically active life, the companionship of my husband, and the company of my friends and family. Fortunately, we are living now in the age of instant access to most information, and I can quickly Google any facts I want to remember. But most of the time, I prefer to exercise my memory by trying to recall the information I want on my own. Unfortunately, my recall has become much slower as I grow older.

Let me give you some examples of my common, frustrating, but not disabling memory problems that become more frequent for most people as we age, especially after the age of sixty-five. Certain seldom-used words are always difficult for me to remember (symbiotic, for example); fortunately, they aren't the words I most commonly use. Particular acronyms like IED have been hard for me, as I struggle to recall what the letters stand for. (I could get "explosive devices," but what on earth was the I for? Finally, it would come to me: "improvised." That was the most common use, but it was an innocent word that never seemed to fit the lethal nature of the weapon.) Sometimes, when trying to think of a Spanish word, I experience what is called "negative transfer," where a French word learned earlier comes to mind—and to lips—first.

I also have the common experience of time delay when, after giving up trying to remember something, the answer comes to mind on its own sometime later, even much later. (Last night, after a discussion about poetry, I tried to remember the name of T.S. Eliot's famous poem. When I opened my eyes this morning, the first words to literally pop into mind were *The Waste Land*, leaving me to wonder again about memory and the philosopher René Descartes's theories on brain-mind duality.) And then, proper names sometimes either leave my mind a blank, or leave me unable to fill in my mnemonic memory aid of recalling initials or first letters (for example, a woman in our church looks like the actress Juliette Binoche, but sometimes I'd remember instead Jacqueline Bisset, and after my brain had already made one JB connection, any other one wasn't forthcoming). For many of us, the loss of nouns—that is, the names of people and things—is the most annoying. These examples and many others make me worry and complain about my memory, even if what I experience is still in the category of age-associated normal forgetting.

The brain—that three-pound, twin-lobed, wrinkled reservoir of our knowledge—comprises only about 2 percent of one's body weight, but uses 25 percent of one's glucose energy as well as 20 percent of one's total oxygen consumption. In fact, 20 to 25 percent of one's blood goes to the brain. (When you're thinking hard, the brain may use up to 50 percent of your fuel and oxygen.)

Whether we're learning or remembering, storing or retrieving, the chain of events is the same. The brain is composed of some one hundred billion specialized nerve cells called neurons. Each neuron has a sending end, the axon, and a receiving end, the dendrite. A neuron's axon, coated in a fatty substance called the myelin sheath, sends an electrochemical impulse away from the cell's body across a gap, or synapse, to the receiving, dendrite end of another neuron. Once the dendrite picks up the signal, it relays it to its neuron's axon to be transmitted to the next cell body, and so on. Each transmission from one neuron to another is aided by a neurotransmitter such as serotonin, dopamine, GABA, norepinephrine, glutamate, or acetylcholine. Glutamate, the most common neurotransmitter, strengthens the synaptic connections. Acetylcholine is particularly critical for memory and learning; it also supports communication between brain cells, but drops dramatically to about 10 percent as dementia progresses, in spite of anticholinergic drugs like Aricept. All together, this is the cellular basis for thoughts, memories, sensations, and emotions.

Just as our body ages, the brain itself goes through changes triggered by inflammation, allergens, foods, toxins, and stress. Beginning at age twenty, we slowly begin to lose neurons, and by the age of seventy-five, nearly one-tenth of the neurons we were born with have shrunk or died due to disease. The mitochondria—the energy factories of the cells—begin to be destroyed, and without them, neurons can't turn glucose into energy. Amyloid plaques form. The myelin sheaths that protect nerve fibers may fray, reducing the level of neurotransmitters and disrupting the normal timing in neuron circuits. Memory slows down. Thus, so-called "normal forgetting" is often due to the loss of speed in cognitive processing that comes with age. When we can't remember something we know, it's because the connection between neurons has been disrupted.

Could it also be that, in addition to biological changes, the cumulative effect of years of learning, of assimilating more and more information, means that the aging brain just needs extra time to search for and find what one wants and bring it to consciousness? This has long been one of my favorite pet theories, more so as I'm older. I used to imagine the brain stretching like a rubber band, not to the point of snapping, but taking longer to make connections along its increased size. But in a recent study, Dr. Michael Ramscar in Germany instead compared the brain to a computer. When the computer was loaded with more information until it had a filled-up hard drive, he found that just like a healthy brain, the computer became slower. "The human brain works slower in old age," Dr. Ramscar says, "but only because we have stored more information over time."[11]

How much more information? We continue to form and add more connections as we accumulate new information throughout our lifetimes. The estimate is that each of our 100 billion neurons may be connected to as many as 10,000 other neurons, with signals going through as many as 1,000 trillion connections or synapses, as many as 125 trillion in the cerebral cortex alone. The human brain was once said to mirror the number of stars in the Milky Way. "As above, so below," Hermes Trismegistus mused centuries ago, and that was long before the invention of modern telescopes. Now, in the universe of Hubble, scientists can only estimate within trillions the number of stars in the billions of galaxies. A more accurate comparison to the brain may be the equivalent of a computer with about a trillion gigabytes, or 75 billion 16-gigabyte iPads. The wonder isn't that some connections misfire. The miracle, and the awe, is that so many of them succeed.

One more part to consider before we know how what is "out there" (i.e., in the world around us) gets to be "in here" (in our head, our mind, our brain) is the coordination of the process. We think of memory as residing in the brain, especially in the hippocampus, but in fact, the hippocampus is more like the conductor of a symphony. The sensations of an experience come from many different parts of the brain: the occipital lobe records visual perception; the amygdala, our sense of smell; the auditory cortex, sound; and so on. All of these sensory impulses are then sent to the hippocampus, which coordinates them into a singular composition and records them. Just like a symphony, however, slight variations may occur when the memory composition is played back. Over time, what we remember may be what we *remember* that we remember. Is it any wonder that each person's perception of an event may be slightly different from that of another observer? Or, that eyewitness accounts may contain contradictory testimonies according to the perceptions registered? Reality doesn't consist of one completely true objective version that everyone agrees on. Phenomenology reminds us that reality is subjective, what we perceive to be true. (Also, think of Heisenberg's Uncertainty Principle in quantum physics. For example, regarding whether light is a wave or a particle, we can know with precision *either* the position (particle) or the momentum (wave), depending on how we set up our experiment. In other words, we "know" the reality we perceive by the way we choose to look.)

Furthermore, memory has four different levels. First, the sensory level comes from various areas of the brain, as described above. For example, we remember visions (called iconic memory), a pretty melody (echoic memory), or a favorite aroma of chocolate chip cookies baking. Some of these memories are fleeting and fade quickly, but others can be very long lasting, especially those of smell, since the olfactory cortex is located close to the hippocampus and amygdala. Even our skin and muscles may hold sensory memories that can be evoked years later through certain massage techniques like bioenergetics. The second level is the working memory, primarily involving the prefrontal cortex that governs attention, concentration, and short-term retention such as keeping a phone number you've just heard in mind until you need it or can write it down; then it's forgotten. But if you hold on to that information longer, you store it in the third level, short-term memory. Once short-term memory fails, as it does for Alzheimer's patients, then no more new memories can be added to the fourth level, long-term memory. But long-term memory will continue to exist for a while after short-term memory fails and may be accessible without receiving anything new. Eventually, though, with Alzheimer's, most of it, too, will be wiped out.

It's one thing for an Alzheimer patient not to remember what was said a few minutes ago. It's a very different thing not to remember the past. Long-term memory holds many different types of memories, each a unique kind of experience. Some are called implicit or procedural memory for actions that may become effortless or even unconscious after many repetitions, like how to drive a car or how to play the piano. (Maurice Ravel, in spite of having Alzheimer's disease, remembered how to conduct his orchestral composition *Bolero* and continued to make recordings every year until his death.) As in Ravel's case, such automatic memories, stored in the cerebellum, can remain intact much longer. Explicit memory requires more conscious effort before it's moved into long-term memory where it's further divided into either episodic (sequence and time, such as, "I moved to California before I went to graduate school") or semantic (consisting of general knowledge, recognition of names or objects, and facts, such as an isosceles triangle has three equal sides).

Of all these types of memories, episodic, processed and organized by the hippocampus, is the part of memory that holds the individual stories we tell ourselves over and over again until they become our identity. Aristotle called memories "the scribe of the mind," and your episodic memory is your autobiography. Tragically, episodic memory, the very story line of your life and who you are, is the first part of long-term memory to be destroyed by Alzheimer's. Identity becomes confused, then it may disappear completely, and the patient is lost in a crowd of unknown persons occupying the brain.

\*\*\*

Knowing what was going on in my mother's brain was obviously impossible and could be guessed only from clues in her behavior. I do know that she wasn't complaining about her memory. By this stage, at the age of eighty-eight, she never mentioned its loss, usually a sign of memory impairment. And she definitely had bad memory days. At least once, Mom didn't remember which daughter I was, although she knew I was one of them. I guess that was an improvement over thinking I was her sister.

At other times she could be quite lucid, however, as when she told me at my house, referring to the senior residence, "I'd have to be stupid to want to go back already." Her mental states fluctuated between confusion and clarity, depending on the day and the hour and whether she was alert or tired. These fluctuations are characteristic of early dementia, and the days of clarity give false hope. But neither confused nor clear could be taken to fully describe her level of cognition.

Her behavior as well as her cognitive ability had suffered from her isolation and loneliness during the previous two years, but it, too, fluctuated. With social interaction and stimulation she could be much better—at times. While she was at our house, I tried my best to bring joy and happiness into her life by revisiting the activities she used to enjoy. Ed and I took her to movie theaters twice. I took her to a beauty shop once and washed and set her hair the other times myself. We went to restaurants, went shopping at the large, outdoor Stanford Shopping Center (where I helped her buy a pair of shoes), and went on short walks. We watched more old movies and cable TV—she especially liked the 1954 movie *Young at Heart* with Doris Day and Frank Sinatra. We listened to Mozart, who used to be her favorite classical composer, while we baked cookies. We also had a few family gatherings, including a rather large extended-family party of sixteen people on Mother's Day. She enjoyed the attention, and we took a photo of the four generations of females in my family. In the front row are my daughter Renée, her daughter Audrey, and Mother. Standing behind, I'm holding a photo of Claire (my son Mark's daughter who lives in Connecticut); next are my daughter Karen and her daughter Lauren.

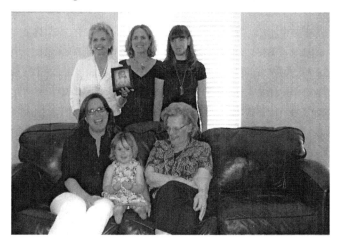

Mom was delighted again and delightful; she was engaged in living. The contrast in her behavior at our house compared to when she was living among strangers can be described very simply. As rigid and stubborn as Mom could be in her own environment, once outside of it she improved and was able to participate in activities and even enjoy herself. For example, the day Ed and I had arrived in Nevada to pick her up, she refused to go out to a restaurant for dinner with us and instead slipped across the hall to the dining room. In contrast, while visiting us in California, she had no problem going out with us to new places or even staying alone at times (the day we had matinee opera tickets, she took a nap and then waited for our return). Before leaving to go back to the residence center, she was helping to set the table and do the dishes, even emptying the dishwasher when I wasn't at home.

Our experience with her was like watching a flower begin to bloom. She once or twice asked Ed to pour her a drink of Scotch before dinner, something she used to enjoy. She liked eating the favorite ethnic foods that she used to cook. She loved having company, hugs, physical contact, and the comfort of a companion. (She still had to be coaxed to take a daily shower, but she could do so on her own.)

Yet toward the end of this or any previous visit to our house, Mom would seldom want to stay longer than two weeks before she began to worry, saying, "I need to get back." When I asked her why, I learned that she thought she had a family somewhere waiting and expecting her to return; "they" needed her and she'd be "missed." This had been true for so much of her life. Now she couldn't remember where she lived or who these family members might be.

"Who needs you, Mom?" I'd ask.

"Michael," she'd say, but this was an ambiguous answer since both my father and my brother were named Michael. At least she knew a name; perhaps she meant both of them.

I typed a sheet of paper in large print and mounted it on cardboard for her to see her address in Nevada and where each of us lived in relation to her so she could consult it whenever she was confused. (I included our names and phone numbers, but she never could call us from the phone in her room.) Here's the sign I made for her:

My name is Madeline Emma.

I was born on March 2, 1920. I'm now 88 years old.

I live in a senior residence in Nevada. I have a studio apartment, number —. I've lived there on my own since May 2006.

My husband Michael passed away in January 2005.

My son Michael and his wife Agnes live nearby. He's a medical doctor.

My daughters Kate (husband George) and Patricia (husband Wallace) live in Southern California, about a four-hour drive from where I live.

My daughter Connie (husband Ed) lives in northern California, about a nine-hour drive from where I live.

My family members call me and visit whenever they can.

I can go and visit them for as much time as we agree on.

Where I live, I have an aide who comes in the morning to give me my pills and help me.

I eat three meals a day in the dining room there.

As the time drew closer to take her back to Nevada, I tried to visualize what my own future might be like. Would I be shuffled back and forth from one of my children to another, with no memory, no judgment, no clear mind? Would they be dreading to see me come and happy (or at least relieved, as I sometimes was now with my mother) to see me go? And perhaps feeling guilty either way?

On Monday May 12, 2008, I flew with her to the Las Vegas airport and escorted her back by cab to her lonely room. Initially she said she didn't remember this place, but she seemed to adjust to it very quickly. We ate lunch, and she helped me to unpack her clothes. As I was leaving she asked me, "Will I ever see you again?"

*** 

After Mother's visit with us I wrote Michael a description of her behavior at our home, and I told him about a seminar on memory loss and Alzheimer's disease Ed and I had just attended that previous weekend. The neurologist and psychologist on the UCSF faculty, both with impressive credentials, listed various causes for diverse types of dementia and stated that Alzheimer's, the most frequent type of dementia, is a disease and isn't necessarily a part of aging (a fact worth repeating many times to reassure our population of aging baby boomers). Since clinical tests can now determine Alzheimer's disease with 90 percent accuracy, the speakers said, there's a need for a full clinical evaluation because Alzheimer's should be correctly diagnosed and treated. Different disorders of the brain require different interventions, and a lot of changes in treatment have developed in the past five years, we were told. Also, the patient needs to have a complete physical screening to first rule out any organic causes, such as a $B_{12}$ deficiency. Because I hadn't received any of this information, I asked my brother what clinical tests Mom had had.

Without criticizing him, I shared my belief that social deprivation was and is a huge factor in her regression and that social stimulation is vitally critical to her. Her brief time with the visiting angel wasn't sufficient for her needs because after the aide left, Mom would just go to her meals and spend the rest of the day sitting on her couch or sleeping. Even our visits, whether half an hour, two hours, or even two full days, weren't sufficient. In my estimation after our experience, Mom needed longer and more frequent visits away from the senior residence. I suggested that even if she couldn't remember who was with her or what we did, at any present moment she could be much happier if we all tried to make Mom's life more pleasant.

Michael wrote back to me:

> To bring you up to date over the past nine years here in Nevada, she has seen three internists (if I count myself as one), two neurologists, and a clinical psychologist for evaluations, and they have diagnosed her with Alzheimer's-type dementia. She has been on medications for this for years, and [it] seems to be keeping her from rapidly progressing. She has a

podiatrist...and a home care nurse that comes daily to give her medications and perform hygiene. She does get very stubborn with them and I try to encourage her to allow them to help her, putting the blame for the aid on her arthritis, as discussing her memory makes her more frustrated.

She has had many lab tests that have been run; her thyroid level is fine, and all other treatable causes for dementia have been ruled out. The MRI scans show temporal lobe atrophy bilaterally and white matter small vessel changes. I'm glad you and Ed attended a program regarding dementia, but I assure you all avenues have been tried with specialists' care.

...She's there so she can socialize, as my wife and I both have full-time jobs. I call her and try to get her to go socialize; I go there and try to introduce her to new people. Often we go to visit her on weekends...I ask Mother if she wants to go to dinner or go out for dessert or just go see a casino, etc., but she's very resistant and refuses. Often I have to argue just to get her to take a shower, wash her hair, and put on clean clothes.

Mother is there because of how poorly she was doing by herself while I was at work. She didn't eat or even drink fluids while alone, and it became a dangerous situation. The clinical psychologist felt she'd do better if she had social interactions at an assisted living facility. I think overall it has helped maintain some independence over the past few years, but she's becoming more reclusive and stubborn. She has good days and bad days, or should I say moments to moments?

I answered:

My letter was meant to inform, not to criticize anyone. I believe that our mother completely devoted herself to all of us while we were young. But after two years, in spite of everyone's best intentions, I think that her situation is less than ideal. I'm not sure that those who are being paid to care for her are doing enough.

I do appreciate your bringing me up to date. I was never informed of her exact diagnosis or the number of tests that she had. With my background, I'm aware of the different areas of the brain and the functions that they control. Certainly I suspected that she had an early stage of Alzheimer's, although she could have had another type of dementia or been affected by other physical causes.

Although I wasn't a part of either the original decision to move her from your house or the choice of placement for her, I certainly agree that it wasn't good for her to be alone all day while you worked. Nor do I think she should be alone all day now.

My point is that outside of her present environment she improves and is able to participate and enjoy herself. I'd like to see her have more breaks away from there, being with one of us.

One last thought: Given her living conditions, even at our ages, how would we fare?

# CHAPTER FOUR: LOCKED IN

## Alzheimer's Diagnosis, Causes, Myths, and Stages

On Saturday, August 16, 2008, while I was back in western Pennsylvania for my high school reunion, I was eager to visit my special cousin—special because in addition to being my cousin and a classmate, Virginia and her husband had bought my parents' house when they moved to California in 1977. In truth, as much as I loved seeing her, I also loved being in our former house again.

My parents had built the house, hiring subcontractors for most of the work, but doing what they could on their own. I remember my mother, eight months pregnant, varnishing bedroom and closet doors just before we moved in. She gave birth to my sister Kate shortly after (at that time, prenatal toxins weren't widely discussed; fortunately, Kate wasn't harmed). The house was a 1950s-style one-story brick ranch house, centered on a large lot in a newly developed area on the single hill of our small town in western Pennsylvania. Behind our property was a wooded area and space for a large garden that I helped weed, among my other chores. I wasn't quite ten years old when we moved in, and after I went away to college eight years later, I never really lived in that house anymore. But I have so many memories of my years there.

Seeing it again was like visiting a place known from a dream—similar in form, yet different in detail. I thought it would be great to call my mother and let her know I was standing in her former kitchen. Maybe the image might spark some memory of the past where she'd spent so many years and where her children had grown up. Maybe it would make her happy to picture me there.

But no one at the senior residence knew where Mom was.

"Try calling the beauty salon," the receptionist who answered the phone suggested to me. I had my doubts because, even though the salon was just down the hall from Mom's room, she seldom had found her way there alone. This time was no exception. She wasn't there.

I tried calling my brother, but since I couldn't reach him, I became quite alarmed that something terrible may have happened to Mom, maybe even a stroke or a heart attack.

After what seemed like endless hours of calls and agonizing worry, I finally reached Michael, who explained what had happened. Mother's usual health care worker had had three days off. When a new aide without a key had come to her door, Mom didn't recognize her voice and wouldn't let her in. Unfortunately, even though August temperatures in Nevada could spike to 112 degrees outside, somehow the air conditioner in Mom's room had been turned off. Whether she'd done this herself or someone had neglected to turn it on, no one knows or will say. What I did learn was that as her room became stifling hot with each passing hour (or day?), Mom had had enough presence of mind to lie down in her underwear on the bathroom floor tiles to cool off. Not one staff member had noticed her absence for an unknown period of time and checked on her, even though she had missed meals.

When Michael found her there at three-thirty on Friday afternoon, the day before my calls, she was both dehydrated and delirious. He called paramedics who rushed her to a hospital, where an internist and cardiologist stabilized her condition; her blood pressure had soared to a systolic reading of 210. An electroencephalogram showed that she had not had a seizure. Four days later, she was still weakened but considered to be well enough to be transferred to a rehabilitation hospital.

The staff at the rehabilitation hospital wasted no time in administering some memory tests to my mother and quickly classified her as definitely having Alzheimer's disease. She was to be transferred to a one-story, locked memory-care unit, the small building alongside the large, two-story main building where she'd been living the past twenty-seven months.

Michael wrote to my sisters and me on August 26, 2008:

> Mother is going to be discharged this coming Saturday. She's unfortunately going to have to change apartments to the secured unit in the back, which is locked, with a twenty-four-hour attendant. She's too confused and wandering around the rehab hospital and not safe on her own, even with a home aide visiting. Her new room will still accommodate most all of her present furniture, but some things will need to be boxed and taken out. She will be in a double room with a roommate because a private room is extremely expensive. We'll also keep a home aide coming that is on her home health policy and no further out of pocket cost; this gives her extra care and attention. The agency is going to be changed to a different one that is in the process of being evaluated.

I responded:

> By "secured unit in the back" are you referring to the memory-care building? When we spoke last week, you were against Mother going there. What happened?

I'm concerned about her "wandering around on her own." This was never mentioned as an issue before. She barely left her room, the dining room, and the lobby. She was reluctant to try the elevator or go up the stairs even with someone to help her. When did things change, and who reported this change? Are they trying to protect themselves from their failure to care for her?

I appreciate your informing us of this possible move, but with all due respect, I'd like to have more discussion and more input. Probably you have good reasons, but I need to know more about them. In short, the thought of her moving is bad enough. To think of her having to spend the rest of her life in a room with another person is intolerable. Once again, I don't want to be challenging, but I'm questioning and needing more information. Let's all think about this together.

Michael replied on August 27:

This decision was made by the rehab hospital and their physicians. Mother actually fell out of bed last night, but no injury, thankfully. Here is the case manager's phone number. They have made the decision, not me and not the administrator where she was living. They state she's not safe and won't allow her to go back to her apartment. I tried to get her to stay where she'd been with more home aide hours, but they refused. She has a "wander bracelet" on so she won't walk out of the building. She doesn't use the walker and is still unstable, but stronger and with very poor recall. The price goes up about $600 a month for the memory care semiprivate room. A private room there costs over $8000 a month. All of the rooms in this unit are kept open door all of the time.

I thanked my brother for the additional information and called the case manager as he suggested. I requested that instead of giving her cognitive tests under these conditions when she was so clearly stressed, she be returned to her studio apartment and given some time to calm down and perhaps regain her pre-accident mental abilities before being tested again. I pointed out that they were making a recommendation based on my mother's behavior in a location that was completely strange to her and where she was bound to be distressed and confused. Everything there was different—people, sounds, smells, food, even having to wear hospital gowns. I suggested it was natural for my mother to be wandering in and out of rooms; she was disoriented and trying to find her room and her own belongings. Also, she wasn't used to sleeping in a single bed, which may be why she'd fallen out of bed the night before. I tried every argument I could think of.

Later I learned from the Fisher Center for Alzheimer's Research Foundation website that dehydration may lead to a false diagnosis of AD, a fact that was repeated at a UCSF conference I attended in March 2014. The speaker at UCSF also added that unfamiliar people, noise, lack of sleep, a strange place, and some medications can all lead to delirium and depression, and that any hospitalization is stressful, especially for individuals with dementia.[12] At the time, however, I simply felt their recommendation in moving Mother now was taking two giant leaps into an irreversible position that was quite possibly more extreme than she needed at her stage.

I also requested that her status where she'd been living be changed from "independent" to "needs assistance." If that had been the case, she never would have been missing because she'd have had someone on the premises to check on her and to help her with basic care such as showering and dressing. "Needs assistance" would have cost more money (although my father had left Mother with an ample amount of money and none of us would've had to cover her costs), but it would have been more secure than depending on the arrival of a visiting angel that the home health-care policy provided.

I wrote to Michael:

> It may very well be that we'll have to make the decision to move her into a memory unit sometime in the future. But I strongly feel that we owe it to her to try a step up first before we do something that could really put her over the edge of sanity. The case manager told me that you have already found a new home health-care agency that will give Mom three hours a day, which is good; the last one wasn't even giving her one hour. She also said that the decision where Mom lives is up to us, her family, if we are willing to take responsibility for her safety. I for one am completely willing. In fact, I'm even willing to move her to an assisted living facility near me where she can have a private room for approximately $5,000 a month. Please call me when you have time to talk about my idea. Also, I'll be there to see her a week from tomorrow. Please don't move Mom until we can consider all options.

Michael replied that he'd tried to get Mother moved back to her apartment but was informed by the case manager that this wasn't an option. As he pointed out, it certainly was much easier for him if Mom could stay in her own apartment with more care because he wouldn't have to move all her furniture and personal belongings. He added that if he could get agreement for her to return, it would be great, but he'd tried and was met with denial. As he said, "I'm her son in this situation, not the doctor, and not making the decision—just trying to do the best for Mom."

I answered:

> Michael, I'm sure that you're trying to do the best for Mom, not just as her son, but also because you're a doctor and are able to evaluate her present condition.

I'm also trying to be an advocate for her, but obviously I don't have the most recent impressions.

From what you're telling me, she has had a decline in the last two to three weeks. Whether that is the cause or the result of her bad experience with the air conditioner being turned off, we'll never know.

I was waiting to hear back from the nurse at the senior residence to see if Mother could return to her studio apartment, but she never responded to my call. I never heard one word of apology or explanation from the administration about their failure to check on Mother when she was missing at meals, although a simple check of the guest registry would have shown that she'd not been signed out. I suspect that the decision not to take her back had as much to do with their refusal to accept future responsibility as it did with the diagnosis of her condition.

Michael wrote to me:

I'd like Mom to stay in her own apartment as well but was getting an absolute "no" answer from the case manager.

I'm very concerned about Mom because she wets her pants and doesn't even know to get them changed. She did this last weekend, and they showed me photos of her scalded skin from urine burns. On top of this, falling out of bed and overall poor balance. When she went to the hospital she had bruises on her knees and ankles in varying stage of healing. This appears to have been going on for a period of time, and Mom has been hiding it.

Equating this last alarming description with the same mother who had visited us for two weeks, including our Mother's Day celebration with her, just three months earlier, was almost beyond my ability to imagine. At that time, she'd been completely continent and had no bruises from falling, nor did she have any burns from scalding or any other causes. What kind of supervision and care had she been receiving? Could she have changed so much so rapidly? Patricia even broke her years of silence and sent me a long e-mail, urging me to "please stop debating this issue." In spite of all the letters and comments, however, I still wasn't clear who was really in charge of the decision.

Nor was I ready to accept the diagnosis of Alzheimer's disease at this point based on whatever tests the staff at the rehabilitation hospital had administered. Had they done the necessary complete blood cell count and blood analyses for levels of vitamin $B_{12}$, glucose, and electrolytes recommended by the American Academy of Neurology? Had they tested thyroid and liver functions? Done depression screening? I doubted very much that they'd checked her biomarkers, although newer studies focus on establishing biomarker criteria and guidelines that will show changes in the brain, cerebrospinal fluid, and blood associated with AD before the symptoms actually appear. My notes indicate that they did perform an MRI that showed "severe atrophy," probably a reference to the bilateral temporal lobe atrophy Michael had only recently told me about, damage that would affect her in many ways. The temporal lobe, which contains the hippocampus, is one of the first brain areas to be damaged by AD. Among other losses for my mother would be the abilities to remember recent events, to recognize faces, and to understand what she hears.

Still, I was suspicious of the diagnosis for good reason. As Dr. Sam Gandy, director of the Mount Sinai Center for Cognitive Health in New York City, says, "One concern about the increased visibility and prevalence of Alzheimer's disease is that some physicians will be tempted to jump straight to that diagnosis without first having followed the 'rule out reversible causes' rule.'" He adds, "We must always seek to exclude treatable, reversible causes of dementia such as depression, nutritional deficiencies, endocrine disorders, and metabolic disorders before rushing into a diagnosis of Alzheimer's."[13]

\*\*\*

Why was I resisting "a diagnosis of Alzheimer's" for my mother? I resisted because Alzheimer's isn't treatable or reversible, but dementia may be. Dementia is defined as a significant decline in mental ability that persists over time in two or more categories: memory loss, language, reasoning and judgment, visual perception, and ability to focus and pay attention. Dementia causes problems, it's true, but some hope exists with certain types of dementia.

According to Dr. Peter Rabins, dementia can be treated and reversed in about 1 percent of cases.[14] Only by ruling out the following *reversible* or treatable causes of dementia is a diagnosis of Alzheimer's then considered to be 90 percent accurate. These include:

- hypothyroidism,
- depression,
- an operable brain tumor,
- vitamin-$B_{12}$ deficiencies,
- drug and alcohol abuse,
- sleep disturbances, and
- toxic reactions to either prescription or over-the-counter drugs, especially sleeping pills.

Many dementias, on the other hand, are *irreversible* and come from a variety of other causes, such as:

- Alzheimer's disease (accounts for about 70 percent of cases),
- vascular dementia (accounts for about 17 percent of cases),
- frontotemporal dementia,
- dementia with Lewy bodies,
- Down syndrome,
- AIDS,
- Huntington's disease,
- Parkinson's disease,
- Pick's disease,
- Creutzfeldt-Jakob disease, and
- brain disorders caused by trauma, illness, and infection.

In spite of its prevalence in this group, diagnosing Alzheimer's disease has been problematic ever since the German doctor Alois

Alzheimer first reported brain abnormalities in his fifty-one-year-old female patient, Mrs. Auguste D., in 1906. Certainly, she wasn't the first person ever to show debilitating memory loss; many famous people throughout history who'd lived long lives eventually suffered with what became known as "senile dementia" because of its association with old age. But Mrs. Auguste D. was a special case that attracted widespread attention, not only because of her relatively young age, but because Dr. Alzheimer's report on her autopsy described damage he'd never before seen: shrinkage of the brain's cortex that is involved in memory, thinking, judgment, and speech. He also described "clumps," now known as amyloid plaques, and "knots" or "neurofibrillary tangles," now called "tau," throughout her brain. The publication that described his findings gave his name to the disease.

The rather pejorative term "senile," however, was still used throughout the 1940s and continued the false belief that cognitive decline was a part of normal aging caused by cerebral arteriosclerosis. Then in the 1950s, technical advances such as electron microscopes allowed researchers to study the structure of the brain and see the plaques and tangles directly related to Dr. Alzheimer's discovery a half century earlier. The term "senile" was dropped when it was recognized that younger persons from thirty to fifty years old, like Mrs. Auguste D., could also have "Alzheimer's disease" as it is now called. Often abbreviated and used interchangeably with AD, Alzheimer's disease was recognized as a distinct disease and its diagnostic criteria were first outlined in the *Diagnostic and Statistical Manual of Mental Disorders* in the 1980s.

Then in 2002, a UCLA research team discovered a new way of using positron emission tomography (PET) that showed in living patients the same kind of tiny plaques and tangles Dr. Alzheimer had first seen under a microscope after his patient died. Plaques, which look something like fried eggs, are made of a protein called beta-amyloid that blocks cell-to-cell communication between neurons at the synapses and may also activate immune system cells, triggering inflammation there. Tangles are also composed of a protein, this one called tau. Tau resembles parallel strands like railroad ties that support the vital cell-transport system of nutrients within the neuron. When tau collapses into twisted neurofibrillary threads or tangles, nerve-cell death results. Today's researchers are largely either the "baptists," who research beta-amyloid plaques, or the "tauists," who consider tau to be a more primary cause of Alzheimer's, and the two groups compete for scarce research dollars.

Based on MRI imaging of memory changes in major brain regions, scientists at Columbia University Medical Center say that Alzheimer's begins in the temporal lobe at the lateral entorhinal cortex (LEC), the gateway to the hippocampus where new learning takes place and memories of recent events are formed. It progresses eventually to other areas of the cerebral cortex, especially the parietal cortex that is involved in spatial orientation and navigation. Sensory functions of vision and smell become impaired, and personality may change. Neurons break down structurally with beta-amyloid plaques and tau tangles, and the cholinergic neurons produce less of the neurotransmitter acetylcholine so critical for learning and memory. The brain becomes riddled with holes as the four ventricle cavities filled with cerebrospinal fluid expand and the cortex shrinks in size. This is *what* happens, but it doesn't explain *why* it happens. Several theories exist, but none so far are conclusive and incontrovertible.

One difficulty of diagnosis is that the presence of beta-amyloid plaques and/or tau neurofibrillary tangles in a PET scan is not necessarily predictive of Alzheimer's disease. Even if both are present, an individual may have no cognitive deterioration; about one person in five receives a mistaken false positive diagnosis. Among twenty-one subjects with mild cognitive impairment whose PET scans showed plaques and tangles spread throughout several regions of the brain at the beginning of a study, only six individuals (29 percent) were diagnosed with Alzheimer's during follow-up two years later.[15]

Still unknown, therefore, is whether plaques and tangles are the cause or the effect of Alzheimer's disease. Some researchers are now looking beyond the structural damage they cause in the brain, focusing instead on the functional interaction and communication between brain regions, such as the prefrontal cortex and hippocampus, affected by the decline in neurotransmitters. Other researchers are pursuing different theories: Is AD a prion (infectious protein) disease? Or is Alzheimer's caused by a virus? Are plaques really the result of tiny proteins called oligomers that are toxic to brain cells? Does chronic inflammation destroy neurons? Or are neurons destroyed by free radicals that cause oxidative stress? Do the imperceptible ministrokes called microinfarcts that are common in older adults contribute to dementia?

With no full knowledge of how and why Alzheimer's disease begins, a number of early theories were advanced. All of these have now been relegated to the category of myths, according to the Alzheimer's Association:

- **Myth**: Memory loss is a natural part of aging.
  **Fact**: AD is a disease that causes brain cells to malfunction and die.
- **Myth**: Alzheimer's disease isn't fatal.
  **Fact**: No one survives AD.
- **Myth**: Only older people can get AD.
  **Fact**: AD can strike people as young as thirty years old.
- **Myth:** Aluminum, aspartame, flu shots, and silver dental fillings can all increase the risk of AD.
  **Fact**: None of these have been confirmed to be true.
- **Myth:** Treatments are available to stop the progression of AD.
  **Fact**: Not at this time.

***

As it stands now, since a definitive diagnosis for Alzheimer's disease can't be made until autopsy, I was still not completely certain that my mother had AD at this time, especially since I'd recently spent two weeks with her and observed her behavior closely every day. But given the fact that most of the causes for reversible dementia had been ruled out in my mother's case, I had to concede that she would probably have Alzheimer's disease eventually because it's the most prevalent of the irreversible dementias, and she did have certain risk factors.[16]

- First, of course, was her **age**, eighty-eight years old. Alzheimer's disease is still correlated with old age—again, age doesn't cause AD, but the risk of having it increases with age. According to the Alzheimer's Association, beginning at age sixty-five, the risk of developing Alzheimer's doubles every five years. At that age, the chance of developing dementia in one's remaining lifetime is one in twenty. Thirty-two percent of those aged eighty-five have AD; after that, the risk of developing it reaches nearly 50 percent.
- Being f**emale** also puts her at higher risk. Because more women are in the older age groups, and because women live longer with dementia than men do, almost two-thirds of AD patients are women. After the age of sixty-five, roughly 3.2 million women have AD, compared to 1.8 million men. In terms of percentage, past the age of seventy-one, 16 percent of women have AD; 11 percent of men do. Some researchers continue looking for a hormone effect with the decrease of estrogen after menopause, but none has been substantiated so far.
- In terms of **education and socialization**, Mother had only an eighth grade education and hadn't challenged herself intellectually. She socialized mainly with her own family. Women with higher education are 45 percent less likely to develop dementia compared to women with less education.

On the positive side, however, Mom's risks were lower because she:
- smoked rarely, if ever,
- drank little alcohol,
- maintained a healthy weight and an adequate diet,

- married, and
- had good exercise and sleep levels.

Also she did not have two other risk factors:

- Stroke or head injury
- Diabetes

Clearly, however, my mother already did have some stage of dementia (now also called "neurocognitive disorder"). My brother, a medical doctor, saw Mother's condition in terms of symptoms and a disease that needed medication. I saw her in psychological terms as a person troubled by loss of memories and cognitive impairments, but still an individual with abilities and emotions that existed in spite of those losses.

*** 

At what point then do memory problems become dementia? There is a continuum of memory and cognitive problems that ranges from the first two stages of normal, preclinical changes called Age Associated Memory Impairment (AAMI) and Age Associated Cognitive Decline (AACD), to Mild Cognitive Impairment, and then on to stages of dementia. Many diagnostic settings use the rating scale developed in 1982 by Dr. Barry Reisberg, the Clinical Director of New York University's Aging and Dementia Research Center, to help determine the progression of neurocognitive disorder.[17] The stages in Reisberg's rating scale are numbered in order of increasing severity, and they may overlap. Also, not everyone who is in one of the earlier stages will go on to develop later symptoms on the continuum. The website Alz.org has an expanded description of these stages:

- **Stage one**: No impairment
  Normal function: The person does not experience any memory problems. An interview with a medical professional does not show any evidence of symptoms.
- **Stage two**: Very mild cognitive decline (affects half the population over the age of sixty-five). May be normal

age-related change or very early Alzheimer's. Stage two is a critical stage when early intervention can be most effective.

- **Stage three**: Mild cognitive decline (MCI): poorer memory than usual for age, serious enough to be noticed by patient and others, but not serious enough to interfere with Activities of Daily Living or functioning independently.

  MCI is considered to be a stage of transition between normal aging and mild dementia, affecting 10 to 20 percent of people age sixty-five and older. Although MCI does not always lead to dementia, up to 15 percent of those with MCI will progress to Alzheimer's disease each year, compared to 1 to 2 percent of the general population.[18] One out of every two people with MCI will develop AD within three or four years—but 50 percent will not.

- **Stage four**: Moderate cognitive decline (early stage Alzheimer's disease)

  Some difficulty with Activities of Daily Living, such as bathing

  Anxiety, depression, or agitation may be present

  Trouble with trivial activities

- **Stage five**: Moderately severe cognitive decline

  Needs help with Activities of Daily Living, such as dressing

  First stage of obvious dementia

  Problems remembering autobiographical data (address, phone number) and major life events

  Family members may not be recognized

  Problems with sleeping and wandering

- **Stage six**: Severe cognitive decline (middle dementia or moderate Alzheimer's)

  Cannot perform basic Activities of Daily Living, including feeding

  Weight loss

  Noticeable personality changes

  Loss of bladder and bowel control

- **Stage seven**: Very severe cognitive decline
  Communication and motor impairment; may not be able to speak or walk
  Totally helpless and dependent on others
  May comprise 40 percent of the time living with AD

Although the above scale provides a guide, Alzheimer's disease doesn't present the same symptoms, behaviors, or progression for each individual, and stages aren't always clearly delineated until the final ones. In contrast to my mother, one of our friends, a brilliant attorney and head of a large successful law firm, moved very quickly from some symptoms of memory loss and confusion, to needing a round-the-clock caretaker at home, to full-time residential care, to being unable to recognize even his wife, all within the space of a few years. He died in his mid-seventies.

My mother at the time of her hospitalization after the air conditioning incident did not show the behavioral symptoms of irritability, anxiety, or depression sometimes seen in early stages of AD. Her symptoms were a combination of mild cognitive decline (MCI), stage three, overlapped somewhat with parts of stages four and five. Memory was her chief problem, but she could dress herself and could recognize family members. She still had basic skills that I wanted to help her maintain for as long as possible. And Alzheimer's disease was so much worse than her present condition. Memory losses due to aging, those so-called "senior moments," are mischievous kittens of forgetfulness compared to the ravenous tiger of Alzheimer's that slowly devours the brain and the very essence of selfhood. My mother's current stage was more analogous to that of a pet cat.

AD has been considered by many to be a fate worse than death. Alzheimer's disease slowly deteriorates not just memories but also one's identity and sense of self. The very processes of thinking, judgment, and problem solving disappear as brain cells stop functioning, lose connections, and die. Over time, the brain—especially the hippocampus and prefrontal cortex—shrivels and shrinks.

Although the rate of progression varies from person to person, the path is unrelenting. AD leads painfully from loss of memory to the inability to communicate with others, to a loss of basic self-help skills like eating and continence, to possible delusions or hallucinations, and even to personality changes. Gradually the person becomes bedridden and helpless, unresponsive to surroundings and unable to recognize family and loved ones. Eventually, there is susceptibility to other illnesses, pneumonia being the most common, as the motor system that governs swallowing and breathing deteriorates, leading to death. As Harry Johns, president and CEO of the Alzheimer's Association says, "Unfortunately, today there are no Alzheimer's survivors. If you have Alzheimer's disease, you either die *from* it or you die *with* it."

***

Is there any wonder I resisted the diagnosis and preferred that my mother be classified with MCI, which doesn't always lead to Alzheimer's? Placing my mother in a memory-care unit among a group of Alzheimer's patients was to consign her to their same fate too soon, I thought. Nevertheless, my protests were in vain. The decision had been made. Mother was being moved to a new residence for the second time in twenty-seven months, surely a source of more disorientation, confusion, and possibly depression for her.

September 1 was four days away, and Michael and Patricia wanted Mom to be moved into the memory-care unit before the month began. Her queen-sized bed, a nightstand, a chair, a small cabinet, and a TV with stand were squeezed into her new quarters—a hospital sized room with two beds (separated by a curtain and later a partial wall) and a shared bathroom. She and her roommate also shared the one sliding-door-type closet. It had space for hanging clothes at either end and, in the middle, two shelves apiece for folded clothes. Shoes went below, and larger items like extra blankets could be stored on the shelf above. Mother's remaining wardrobe was reduced to a bare minimum; not even one warm coat was in her closet. Evidently, no one was planning to take her outside for a while. (I took her a warm coat.)

With regard to her roommate, Patricia and I had both been wrong. Far from bonding together and becoming new friends, as my sister had thought, the two women never even spoke to one another. Nor did my mother seem to mind sharing the room with a stranger, as I'd predicted. It may have been because my mother's roommates usually spent almost all of their time in bed, sleeping.

In spite of the limited space and loss of her privacy—as well as almost everything else Mom had once owned—I tried to have a positive attitude about the possible advantages of memory care as I found them there. The staff (all but two were female) was attentive and kind. Since the number of residents varied, it was difficult to determine a resident-staff ratio, but usually there seemed to be at least thirty residents at any given time; the maximum number was forty. Almost all were elderly females; just a few were older men. Most of them probably had late-onset Alzheimer's, sometimes abbreviated as LOAD.

Two younger women in the memory-care unit had the rare early-onset form of Alzheimer's disease that strikes before the age of sixty. One of them, an attractive woman with long dark hair, perhaps in her late forties, spent long, lonely hours in an otherwise empty sitting room, staring at the moving shapes on the television. This cruel form of AD accounts for about 5 percent of Alzheimer's patients, or currently about two hundred thousand individuals; by 2050, up to sixteen million people may be afflicted with early-onset AD. The exact cause at such a young age is still not known but is believed to be genetic.

The square building was very clean, well furnished, and attractive. A pleasant open-square atrium was in the middle of the locked building so that residents could walk outdoors there (although I never saw any of them take advantage of this), and everything else was arranged around the atrium. On the near, entry side, of the building were reception, the office, a nurses' station, and the dining room. Along the far side of the atrium were the activity area with tables and chairs, an aquarium, a kitchenette for preparing snacks, and an area for watching television. Murals painted on the walls in the activity area portrayed small scenes of the outside world, such as a florist stand, a fruit cart, and a dressmaker's shop window circa the 1940s; recreating an earlier period in their lives has been shown to make people feel and act younger in that surrounding. The patients' rooms were basically arranged on the perimeter along the sides and back of the building.

No particular odors were noticeable. Aside from at mealtime, liquids—even water—weren't available, except for juice offered with a midafternoon snack, and residents were kept in diapers, further eliminating accidents and smells. I don't know if my mother was aware of suddenly having to wear diapers now. Considering Michael's last letter to me, she needed them. Again, this was a rather abrupt, drastic change for her. My brother and his wife kept Mother supplied with those personal needs.

The food was nourishing, varied, and quite good, but the dining atmosphere was beyond dismal. One or two smaller table groups of four managed to hold an occasional conversation, but they were exceptions. One day I counted that of the eight residents at Mother's table, three of them were sleeping and four needed to be fed soft food. My mother, however, ate her meals with gusto. She began a habit of folding her napkin, sometimes with some silverware tucked inside, to carry around with her when she left the dining room. She did the same thing in restaurants, and I had to gently remove the items from her before we left the premises. I think she felt lost without having a purse to carry any longer because when I took her on outings, she often asked me where her purse was.

Best of all, there was a wonderful activity director named Marcos who led seated exercises every morning to stretch the patients' muscles and help their coordination. He devised crafts and games that he personally invited patients to join by going to their rooms and escorting them to the activities. Marcos was an excellent musician and played music from the 1930s and '40s on a keyboard every day, making it sound like a real swing band, encouraging all of the residents to sing along with him. (There is a theory that people become imprinted to the musical genre that was popular when they were about the age of twenty, and that kind of music remains their favorite throughout life.) Even if some of the others just dozed at the activity table or slumped, often drooling, in their wheelchairs, my mother was an enthusiastic and active participant in almost all activities except bingo, especially in her favorite activity, singing along. How interesting that some part of the brain connected to music must also maintain the memory of lyrics! This could be related to the fact that hearing is the last sense to be lost. In fact, some senior residence centers form singing groups composed of their Alzheimer's patients, providing them with an enjoyable activity. Too bad there was no group at this memory-care unit. Mom remembered the words to all of the old songs, and she'd have enjoyed the sing-alongs.

Still, in spite of the level of care, the appearance of the facility, the efforts of the activity director and the visiting angel, the visits from my brother and his wife, my own visits and attempts to stimulate her involvement in the outside world by taking her for outings, my mother continued to decline cognitively in the memory-care unit. I could understand why.

Some things bothered me, even on a daylong visit. Why were the patients denied water to drink throughout the day? I could understand that there were no glasses, but could there not be paper cups available? (I made sure to bring a bottle of water with me to share with Mom after the first time I visited and found it impossible to get any water to drink for myself.) Was withholding water a means of cutting down on diaper changes? Why were activities mostly limited to the mornings? For patients who could no longer read or understand television shows, would the rest of the day not seem terribly boring? With nothing to do all day long, how would anyone stay mentally active?

Seldom did any of the residents initiate a conversation with one another, although they could be quite aggressive and argumentative if someone didn't take turns correctly when they were playing games, such as throwing a foam ball to one another while they were seated around the activity table. As their social inhibitions declined, they also took critical notice and made inappropriate comments about each other's appearances and mannerisms; several made fun of one newcomer who carried around a doll and talked to it as if it were her baby. In many ways, they had regressed to the stage of nursery school children who hadn't yet learned to interact appropriately. My mother unfortunately became one of the ones who would audibly point out odd behavior or appearance, and she wasn't always pleasant to lost souls who wandered into her room. As the years went by, Mom herself might wander into other rooms, not able to find her own.

In time, the staff sometimes referred to Mother as "the walker" because she walked around and around the quad. She'd never been one to sit around and do nothing, and walking was now her only way of staying strong and active. Or perhaps it was just something to do; maybe she missed the walks she used to take when she was allowed to go outside. When the staff requested that she use a walker for balance, she refused and hid the walker under her bed, and when she was placed in a wheelchair, she made sure she got out of it as soon as she was able. When she couldn't sleep, the staff told me, she'd be up at night, walking. Later I learned that wandering or pacing and a change in sleep patterns were two symptoms of the moderate level of dementia. Walking aimlessly is a common sign of agitation, and when not walking, taking naps during the day because of boredom also causes wakefulness at night.

Walking was actually quite good for Mom, however. The exercise helped her circulation and breathing, giving more blood and oxygen to her brain, which improve its functioning. Walking also reduces anxiety, agitation, and restlessness. Yet no matter how long or how fast my mother walked, Alzheimer's was stalking her and gaining ground. In the years she was in the memory unit, she could never, ever outrun it. I finally had to recognize my mother's eventual diagnosis of Alzheimer's disease. She was now almost eighty-nine years old.

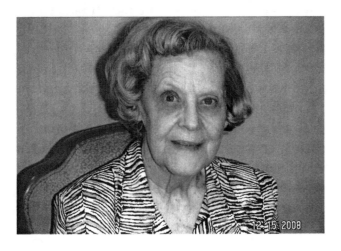

In the memory center where she no longer had her own room, my visits with my mother were mainly day trips—one long day of morning and evening flights plus renting a car at the airport so I could continue taking my mother out to restaurants, shopping, on sightseeing drives, and to movies as long as she was able and willing to go. The first time I tried to sign her out, the office had to call Michael for his permission, which he gave. Perhaps the director was worried I was going to kidnap her after my reluctance to have her moved there. I might have tried, but I didn't have her power of attorney, her medical records, or access to her financial accounts, so there was no way I could move Mother without my brother's permission and cooperation. Nor could I ever bring her with us to Puerto Vallarta again. When I asked him to allow her to come with us on another vacation, Michael said her birth certificate was lost, and he wasn't going to request a new one in order to obtain a passport that the law now required.

Generally, I went alone on my daylong visits to see Mom at the memory center, but sometimes my husband Ed went with me and we'd stay at a hotel nearby to be able to spend two days with my mother. Once, my older daughter Karen accompanied me. Later, my sister Kate and I managed our flight schedules on a few occasions in order to meet each other at the airport in Las Vegas and spend the day together with Mom.

The last movie I was ever able to take Mom to see was, ironically enough, *Mama Mia*. We went to the matinee, which happened to be a sing-along, and we were the only audience in the huge theater. Mom and I held hands, and at the song "Slipping through My Fingers," tears rolled down my cheeks. In the song, the mother is singing to her grown daughter, who is about to leave and begin her own life. For my mother and me, the pendulum of time had swung forward, and our roles were almost the exact opposite of the ones on the screen.

I'm quite sure that as soon as I'd leave Mom and return to the airport for the flight back to San Francisco, she'd forget I'd even come to see her. But if she could be happier for just the few hours of my visit, I knew it was worth my effort to make whatever trips I could. Not only were they making her life more pleasant, they allowed me to spend precious time with her.

Because of the difficulty and expense of visiting her frequently, several times a week I called Mom in the evening for a chat before she went to bed. Patricia had suggested to Michael that he turn off Mother's phone to save money since she wasn't able to initiate calls. He wrote to Kate to ask our opinions, and I explained through Kate why I'd wanted Mom to keep her phone. Fortunately, the phone was never turned off. Those evening talks, sending each other hugs and kisses over the phone, were my way of tucking Mother into bed and wishing her sweet dreams. It was mainly through these evening phone calls that my mother expressed herself the most.

Sometimes when I asked her how her day had been, she'd tell me, "Oh, I was so busy all day." Or, "I went out and did some shopping," or something else she made up. Was she engaging in fantasy to fill her boring days? Was she inventing a story to make me feel good and hide her unhappiness? Or was her lack of stimulation causing her to imagine an alternate reality? Is this what happens to prisoners in solitary confinement?

More often in our conversations, she'd reveal her true feelings about her surroundings. In spite of my eventual, reluctant approval of the memory-care unit for my mother as her needs for help increased, she was never able to accept being there. Over a period of time I kept a record of many of her spontaneous statements because they were so painfully poignant and so full of emotional significance.

The following comments I recorded in shorthand, verbatim from Mother during a long phone call when she was more talkative and ruminative than usual. The time was about nine thirty at night, September 2, 2009, a year and a day after she entered the memory-care unit. I've grouped her comments into the four major themes that concerned her most.

**ESCAPE**

"Everything isn't roses all the time, so then I just told them that I was going to leave."

"I'm still here, and I think I'm just going to go back to my old life. I don't want to be at this place."

"I'll feel better once I get going on my own pattern. Right now I'm just stuck. Once I get myself free, I'll feel much better. I'll redeem myself again. I'll feel more alive again."

**IDENTITY CONFUSION**

"It's something you thought, 'It's what should be,' but it's just different. So I made up my mind it's not the way I want to live. It's not me. You begin to feel like you're nobody. You can't live your life like this, so I just made up my mind to be in my own place."

"It's not anybody's fault. I just lost my sense of right and wrong. I think I took a wrong turn when I came here. I'm just fed up."

"You can't be true to yourself and everybody else. It throws your being right to the core."

"I was happy for a while, but now I'm going to straighten out my whole life like I think it should be. You know, how you felt when you were able to do things, and now you don't feel that way."

"I liked this place, but then I realized it's not my life. I tried it, but it's not what I thought it would be. It's not my life. I did try it, but it's just not me."

**FEAR**

"I'm going downhill kind of fast, and I didn't realize it right away. But suddenly I realized my life was wasted."

"Bit by bit [they] take your life away, wipe you out. [You] go downhill so fast. Down a little at a time, and then I'll be gone."

**HOPE**

"Nobody can tie you down. I made up my mind to do something. I didn't feel like this was what I was supposed to be."

"I'll maybe feel like I'm living again."

"Don't worry about me. This is something I have to figure out for myself."

"Wherever I am, I'll get it all straightened out."

During that entire year, in various phone conversations, Mother often repeated the major themes of escape, identity, and hope, as in these two examples:

"I hope to get home soon. Sometimes I get tangled up in the atmosphere."

"I feel neglected. The more I think about things, the worse I get. I don't feel completely whole. I have to find something or do something just to satisfy myself. It's not as easy as it sounds. The more you start thinking of different things, the worse it gets. You don't satisfy yourself any way. I don't feel like I'm the same person that I was. I've lost it. And now I'm going to actually find it."

By the end of Mom's second complete year in the memory-care unit, the effects of her isolation and lack of stimulation were expressed more in fear and confusion than in hope of escape. Again, in verbatim quotations from her in phone conversations, this is how her downward spiral looked from inside her mind:

### September 30, 2010
"I'm stuck in this house. I have no friends. Don't have anything. I feel so put out. I don't see people I know. It's just a booby trap they [people who put her there] pulled on me."

"I'm wondering where I'm supposed to be. I don't know these people. They're all strange to me. Heck of a way of living. I don't even know what this place is called."

"I've been gone from my place for a while. I feel lost. When I get back to my home, I hope I'll get to see you."

### December 28, 2010
"It's a little scary. I feel like, 'What's wrong with me?' It feels like you're out of it. It feels like you can't control it."

### January and February 2011
"I don't feel good [emotionally]. How much stuff they've taken of mine that I never see again."

"I feel left out of things. I'm left out of everything I had."

"It has to be true. It's been more than one day."

"My hands are tied, too."

"I'm not a necessary person now at all; I feel very unnecessary."

"I don't know how to explain it. They took care of what they thought I needed and that was it. And then they made me sit down and do nothing."

# CHAPTER FIVE: LIGHTS OUT

## Vision Loss and Its Consequences

In June 2011 when I visited my mother, I signed her out of the memory-care unit to take her to lunch at the Italian restaurant we had always enjoyed so much; in fact, this was the same restaurant she and my father had visited the night they became lost nine years earlier. When we entered the dining room, she held back because she said it was too dark and she couldn't see. I thought perhaps her eyes hadn't yet adjusted after coming into a darkened space from the bright sunshine outdoors (dementia patients in particular react strongly to changes in lighting and need moderated brightness), so I guided her across the room to our table by the window where she could see the view of the Las Vegas Strip. But when we left, I wasn't holding her arm tightly enough, and she tripped over the cement parking block in front of my car and fell. Fortunately, she wasn't hurt. I had at least softened her fall.

But because she'd complained about the darkness, when we returned to her room I gave her a cursory eye exam by writing large letters and numbers on a sheet of paper and holding it up before her just a few feet away. She missed identifying most of the symbols. Nor could she recognize my father in the large portrait of his face and shoulders on her wall ("Some woman?" she guessed). This didn't surprise me because once before she'd failed to recognize his photo. As I reflected back, however, for some time I'd been noticing that my mother never wore her eyeglasses anymore, and when I asked Michael's wife, Agnes, about them, she told me that as soon as she replaces them, they're always missing again.

I thought Mother's vision should be checked. Dementia can cause changes in vision that make it difficult to understand what one sees, even differences in colors. Although trouble understanding visual images is one of the ten warning signs that may signal AD, eye exams may be overlooked or considered to be unnecessary. The Singapore Malay Eye Study of 1,032 patients ages sixty to seventy-nine found that those with visual impairment from cataracts or moderate to severe diabetic retinopathy are more likely to experience increasing memory loss and various levels of functional impairment, underscoring the need to effectively diagnose and treat the causes of visual impairment.[19] And although I didn't know it at that time, an Internet report on August 23, 2013, described a study from Cedars-Sinai hospital in Los Angeles that found the amount of beta-amyloid protein in the brain corresponds closely to the amount in the retina in back of the eye. Scientists at Cedars-Sinai are developing an eye test for AD and are starting clinical trials.[20]

I spoke with the director of memory care and asked her if she'd please ask my brother to arrange an eye exam for Mom since I didn't want him to think I was being critical.

"Oh," she told me, "I don't want to interfere. Your brother takes such good care of your mother that I don't like to say anything."

My brother, as I've said, is a physician. He's also the executor of my mother's will and has her power of attorney—mainly, my father had told me, because they were living with him, although I imagine they would have chosen their only son anyway, especially since he's a medical doctor and they felt safe having him oversee their future physical care. In accordance with the HIPPA privacy rules, I don't receive any reports from the memory-care staff since my brother hasn't placed me on the list to be informed about changes in my mother's condition.

I did learn from a cooperative technician, however, that Mom's medications in June included a daily pain pill for arthritis, taken together with a stomach medication on alternate days, as well as thyroid medication and a sleeping pill daily. Considering the side effects and negligible usefulness of memory drugs after a short period of use, I could understand that Mother was no longer taking a medication to delay Alzheimer's effects. She certainly didn't seem to be overly medicated with prescription drugs, although the sleeping pill worried me. Many sleep aids contain diphenhydramine, which suppresses the neurotransmitter acetylcholine—a key brain cell messenger important for memory and learning, as I've stated. Most telling, however, she wasn't receiving any medication for her eyes.

On August 15, 2011 my sister Kate and her husband George went to visit Mother. Kate learned that day from the visiting angel that Mom had been in hospice care the past week after almost a 10-percent weight loss (Mom had weighed a hundred pounds in June but had lost eight pounds in the last two months). Kate also learned from the staff that Mom could see only shadows and had fallen twice because of her loss of vision, but that the family had decided against cataract surgery because of her age (ninety-one) and her mental state. As a result, Mother had to be given total care now and be kept in a wheelchair to prevent future falls.

When Kate called to tell me this news, I was amazed and angry. Why had the director failed to follow up on the eye exam I reported that Mom needed? Why had her vision been allowed to become so much worse in the two months since I'd seen her? I was also extremely upset that neither Kate nor I had been informed about Mother's loss of sight, confinement to a wheelchair, weight loss, and placement in hospice care.

I began to wonder...if Kate had not been there at that time to see Mom's situation, when would she and I have been told about the changes? If I had not tried to call my mother from Pennsylvania three years prior and discovered that she was in the hospital, when would we have been told that she'd been moved to a memory-care unit?

Failure or neglect to provide treatment because of a patient's age or mental condition is a form of elder abuse. To debate this critical issue was to risk further delay in treating my mother, so I turned to the Nevada Elder Protective Services agency for immediate help. They responded quickly and went to speak to the director of memory care even before my husband Ed and I could arrange a visit there the following week.

Prior to our visit I'd called the hospice nurse and the visiting angel and asked them both to meet us at the memory-care unit. When we arrived on September 6, the activity director Marcos was at the reception desk where we signed the visitor registry. He told us that Michael had looked at Mom's eyes and was going to call an eye doctor. We found Mom in the dining room. She was finishing her lunch, eating something soft and sloppy with her fingers since she couldn't see the food (not one of the aides was feeding her as they usually did with other patients who needed assistance). Mom couldn't see us, but she could recognize my voice.

Since neither the visiting angel nor hospice nurse had arrived yet to meet with us, I asked to see Mother's chart. A nurse had to call Michael for permission, which he gave, and he informed the nurse that he was taking Mom to see an eye doctor in ten days.

Her chart showed that she'd been admitted to hospice care on August 8, 2011. At that time her medications were Tylenol for pain, levothyroxine for her thyroid, and trazodone for depression and sleep (at least it didn't contain diphenhydramine). Two weeks later on August 23, two different kinds of eye drops plus medications for arthritis and high blood pressure had been added, and the thyroid medication was changed.

The hospice doctor's intake exam I read stated that my mother has Alzheimer's with dementia, hypertension, arthritis (both rheumatoid and osteoarthritis), depression, and hypothyroidism.

For me, the facts that hypothyroidism was mentioned again and that medication for it was recently changed could be significant. Studies show that for women with either a low or high amount of the thyroid-stimulating hormone TSH, the risk for Alzheimer's disease is increased. The hospice doctor's diagnosis was "debility," and his prognosis for Mother was less than six months of life, based on the facts of depression and not eating. I wondered if she wasn't eating because she couldn't see the food. "She's unable to do most activities and has extensive disease," the report continued. Further information was that an RN could pronounce death and release her body to a mortuary. The "do not resuscitate" order from my brother was dated August 8, 2011. The hospice regulations allowed her to have cataract surgery.

The visiting angel and hospice nurse arrived almost simultaneously. Jean, the visiting angel, said that Mom is the only patient she has ever seen who, in Jean's opinion, has no confusion or fear in her eyes. "She could wear a 'No Fear' T-shirt now. There is no comparison to any patient here," she said. I didn't know whether to be happy that my mother was so calm in facing death or upset at Jean's obvious end-of-life statement.

Stacy, the hospice nurse, said that Mom's dementia was "age related" and that she had high blood pressure. She added that Mother had a loss of interest in food, loss of digestive absorption, loss of ambulation, loss of conversation, and loss of interaction. She also thought that Mom would never be able to walk again, due to losing core strength and having her knees bent for so long in a wheelchair. (Stacy does a full assessment every week or two, and a nurses' aide from hospice comes three times a week.)

She also told us that Michael recently had someone check Mom's eyes and give her eye drops because she has both glaucoma and cataracts. However, Stacy was worried about Mom bending over or pulling out bandages after cataract surgery; she said it was up to the doctor but basically she agreed with Michael and

Patricia's concern about the operation for Mom "because of her age and 'senility.'"

Jean strongly objected to the idea that cataract surgery is dangerous, citing how easy the operation had been in several cases she'd known. I, too, knew from some of my older friends and relatives who had undergone cataract surgery that removing cataracts to restore vision is a very safe and simple procedure for any age person.

Both Stacy and Jean stressed that Mom isn't in distress or frustrated; that she's peaceful, content, and in "her own stage"; that she's a "matter of fact" lady. They would monitor end-stage agitation and give her Risperdal, a tranquilizer for agitation, when necessary. Since my mother had been a faithful Catholic all her life, I requested and they agreed to ask a priest to give Mom the sacrament of the sick. I gave them my phone number and e-mail address but knew they wouldn't call me because of the HIPPA privacy rule.

While I talked with Jean and Stacy in Mom's room, Mom was sitting in her wheelchair outside her door, next to Ed on the sofa in front of the television in the lounge area. He told me later she softly murmured prayers while she moved her fingers as if she were holding a rosary, then made the sign of the cross periodically before she began again to repeat parts of those prayers over and over as a mantra: "Thanks be to God the Father, the Son, and Holy Spirit. Amen," or, "Holy Mary, mother of God, pray for us now and at the hour of our death. Amen," and, "Praise be to God the Father, the Son, and Holy Spirit. Amen."

After Stacy and Jean left, Ed and I wheeled Mom to a quieter area away from the television. All this time, she'd been saying her prayers very softly, and she continued saying them for more than another hour without stopping. I managed at last to have the following conversation with her:

Me: What do you think about when you're praying?

Mom: It's an accomplishment.

Me: Do you mean it's something you have done your whole life?

Mom: I don't remember that.

Me: Well, you learned these prayers as a child, didn't you?

Mom: Yes.

Me: And you said them every night before you went to sleep?

Mom: Yes.

Me: It must be a comfort to you.

Mom: It is.

Me: Isn't it great to know that God is always with you?

Mom: Yes, it is.

Me: Mother, you're a saint, praying for all of us. Are you praying for something?

Mom: Not always.

Me: Just praising God?

Mom: Depends. Different things at different times.

My mother finally had her eye surgery on November 17, 2011, several months after having lost her vision and three months after Kate and George discovered that loss. By chance, Kate and George were on vacation in Las Vegas again for George's birthday the same day of the surgery, and they went to visit Mom at the memory-care facility. Kate later told me that Patricia and Agnes were there and said that if anything had happened to Mom as a result of the surgery, it would have been her fault. They added that they had not intended to allow the surgery except that she (not knowing it was I) had raised "such a fuss." They also told Kate that she could stay and be the one to take care of Mom the rest of the day since they had done enough by taking her to surgery early that morning. Then they left.

Michael's friend, an ophthalmologist, performed the surgery after returning from his vacation. He was able to only remove the cataracts and restore partial sight in Mother's left eye. Since her glaucoma hadn't been diagnosed in time, and treatment not begun soon enough, the glaucoma was too advanced. She remains blind in her right eye.

The surgery itself didn't result in any postoperative problems for Mom, however, and her recovery was very easy. I still cannot understand why my two siblings had refused to provide it.

After Mom's eye surgery, her memory continued to decline. She has a new visiting angel, Beatrice, since Michael and Patricia requested that Jean be replaced after she'd been with my mother for several years. I was sorry to see Jean go. She was a lovely woman who even laundered Mom's personal clothing and linens, hemmed her slacks, framed pictures for her, and found books to read to her about the old movies that Mom loved to watch. The administration at the memory-care unit was also changed (although I don't think this had anything to do with my family). Saddest of all, the excellent activity director is gone now, and the new director leans toward bingo games and bus sightseeing tours of Las Vegas for those who are mobile and more able. On one of my visits there, I saw the activity director sitting with a group of patients at the activity table, reading to them. The only music now comes occasionally from the player piano in the seating area just past the entry. There is no more singing.

Mother is weak now and needs assistance walking, but she still shuns using a wheelchair. Instead, she mostly holds on to railings as she walks around and around the quad. In March 2012, Michael wrote to Kate that Mom was hospitalized with a 104-degree fever and viral pneumonia. As usual, she was a very uncooperative patient, resisting care, pulling out IVs, and refusing food or drink. He wrote, "She declines, especially with dementia and attitude—doesn't want any care right now, but we are trying." No one understood what Mom often had told me, that she preferred to die. Instead, she recovered and went back to walking around the quad.

On two occasions after Mother's eye surgery, Kate and I together took her to restaurants for lunch. Neither of us could have managed the wheelchair, my mother, and the car alone. The first time, which was soon after Mom's surgery, Agnes found us at that same favorite restaurant. We maintained a cordial conversation and didn't mention the eye surgery. The second time Kate and I took

Mom out for lunch was a beautiful day, and we thought she'd enjoy a ride in her wheelchair through some stores in a lovely outdoor shopping center. She did not. The sun bothered her. It was too bright. We gave up and took her into a restaurant for a very early lunch. Only one other table was occupied in our section of the nearly empty restaurant. Still, Mom was covering her head, saying, "Too loud. Too much light." Even the smallest amount of stimulation seemed overwhelming to her now. We hurried through our lunch and brought her back to her room. Our excursions with her outside of the memory-care unit ended that day.

When we returned, Mom took a nap and Kate and I sat on the sofa in the TV area outside of her room while I hemmed the new pair of pants I'd bought for Mom. Later, after Mom awakened, Kate and I moved into her bedroom and were sitting on her bed talking with her when I remembered I'd left my sewing supplies and the pants on the sofa. I went back to retrieve them in the TV area and almost tripped over Patricia, who was standing outside Mom's room with her back to the wall. I hadn't seen her since my father's funeral in 2005. At that time I'd invited her to come to Puerto Vallarta with my mother and us the next day, but she'd declined. Startled at seeing Patricia now, I said, "Oh! Hello." She came into the room to visit Mom with us; her husband soon followed. The conversation was neutral enough until I thoughtlessly mentioned that it was great Mom's eyes were so much better now.

Patricia glared at me and said, "We weren't going to have them done because of the danger."

I glared back and retorted, "How much better it would've been to let her sit blind in a wheelchair until she died." Unfortunately, as in many families, we held totally different opinions and completely disagreed on this very sensitive issue.

My evening phone visits with my mother have almost stopped; she not only doesn't make calls, now she seldom picks up her phone, either. She's especially lucid early in the morning or just after a nap; as she tires, she finds conversation more difficult.

Then, like a stroke victim, she searches for the right words that will not come, so her meaning is often distorted. She has virtually no working memory.

But occasionally I do manage to reach her at one of her good times for a phone conversation. One morning in May 2013 I called her visiting angel Beatrice's cell phone. Beatrice was very dependable and spent a few hours with my mother each weekday morning. I knew I could count on her being there to bring Mom to her room and call me back. I was rewarded with one of the best talks I've had with my mother in some time. She was engaged, connected, and aware. She actually asked me how long she'd been living there. She wanted to know if she ever saw her family anymore, and I told her that she indeed saw all of us whenever we were able to visit. I tried to help her understand that we all still loved her, that we wanted the best for her, and that she was there because that is where she could receive better care. Several times we told each other, "I love you." And then she told me something I will always cherish. "You've always been so good to me," she said.

Her words meant so much to me because I feel I'd failed. I had to admit to myself that there was no way I could have protected my mother from her advancing Alzheimer's disease. By the time Mom's dementia affected her short-term memory to the extent that her memory loss was noticeable to others, the supposed critical window for successful treatment was already closed. Who knew how many neurons had already been lost over that period of several years? But I'd tried my best to slow dementia's advance, to protect her from its worst effects, to recognize her feelings and honor the person that she still is, and to improve her quality of life.

In spite of my efforts, I hadn't saved her from her sense of isolation, from silence, from the absence of stimulation, companionship, love, or even affectionate contact. No wonder that when I call her now I more frequently hear her recent laments:

"Everything is confusing to me. Nothing works like it's supposed to."

"I don't know where everything is all gone to, but it's all gone. That's the way everything goes. My family is completely gone."

"Everything changes everywhere you go. So you have to repattern yourself. It all sounds easy, but it's certainly not easy. When you do get settled down you'll be so happy."

I continue to visit her at least four or five times a year, although when I visited her for her ninety-third birthday, she didn't immediately recognize me because I unfortunately approached her from her side. "Get away!" she snapped. "What do you want?" But as soon as she recognized me, she was fine again, for a while.

She has given up saying the words to her prayers. Instead, she quietly counts to twenty, softly claps her hands twice, makes a sign of the cross, and starts all over again—over and over and over. As I watched her performing this ritual in the dining room, I finally asked her softly if she was afraid of dying. To reassure her, I whispered, "Mother, with all of these prayers, you'll go straight to heaven."

She jumped out of her chair and looked at me with wild eyes. "You go to hell!" she snapped loudly. Even the somnambulant residents around their dinner tables woke up at that. I calmed her down as quickly as I could. This visit was the first and really the only time I'd seen her personality change to aggressive and hostile behavior.

Earlier that day, I'd brought her one of her favorite milkshakes and a sandwich for lunch. Beatrice wheeled her into a separate sitting area where we could have some privacy. After Mom opened the present I brought her, Beatrice and I sang happy birthday to her.

Mom just looked at us. "I'm never happy now," she said.

# CHAPTER SIX: LETTING GO

## Experience of Late-Stage Alzheimer's Disease

Just when we felt certain that Mother would be living out the rest of her days in the memory-care unit, we faced a new development. Kate called on May 20, 2013, to tell me she'd received a text message from Michael: Mom had fallen and broken her right hip and was scheduled for surgery at midnight that same day.

A few days later, when Mother was ready to be released from the hospital, the memory-care unit where she'd been living for almost five years, since August 2008, wouldn't take her back yet; they were afraid of the danger of her falling again since she wouldn't stay in bed. Someone there made the decision to move her by ambulance on May 24 to another hospital in a nearby town for rehabilitation therapy.

I went to visit her in the long-term care unit of the hospital as soon as I could, on June 4. When I arrived, Mom was asleep in a wheelchair at a table next to the nurses' station. Across the table from her was a much younger man, probably in his late forties or early fifties who'd had a stroke and was also in a wheelchair, awake and watching us, but not speaking. I asked the nurses why Mom was there and not in her room. They told me she'd been agitated and was pushing help away that morning, so they'd given her a tranquilizer and wanted to keep an eye on her.

While Mom slept, I talked with both her nurse and the social worker. They were surprised to learn that she had vision in only one eye. I spoke with the physical therapist as well. She explained that the surgeon had replaced just the ball in the hip socket, not the entire hip joint; in her view, this meant a much better prognosis. Mom was already able to put weight on that leg, she reported, and had walked upright between two therapists the day before for about fifteen feet. "That was her first time," the therapist added, "however, she has made impressive progress." Little did she know about my mother's strong drive to be on her feet, walking.

When Mom awoke, she didn't appear surprised to see me. She looked healthy and cared for, except for her hair. But she had manicured nails painted a pale pink, done by an aide as I learned later. A nurse brought her a lunch tray at the table where she was seated in her wheelchair, and I fed her a few bites of pork chop, stuffing, and spinach; she also drank a chocolate-milk booster. Then she refused more food and wanted to lie down.

I was happy to see that she had a nice single, a corner room with a window, at the end of the hall. A lovely pink hydrangea plant, probably from Michael and Agnes, was on the nightstand. Her bed, which she immediately told me she didn't like, has an air mattress with a machine attached to undulate the pressure and prevent bedsores. There were also mattresses on the floor on each side of the bed in case of her falling, and a monitor on her bed to let aides know if she tried to get up on her own. On one side of the bed was her tray stand. She had her own spotless bathroom.

Soon after she lay down, two female aides came into the room to change her diaper. As they moved her, rolling her from side to side in the process, she was resistant and called out to me, "Connie, help me!" Then, "Make them stop, Connie." And again, she called me by name to help her and make them go away. I hadn't told my mother my name that day, nor had she asked me. Considering that she'd been diagnosed with Alzheimer's disease over five years earlier, I was impressed and pleased that not only did she continue to recognize me, she also remembered my name, even under a very stressful situation. Personally, I couldn't even imagine the horror she must have felt at the indignity of having a diaper changed.

After the nurses left her room, she fell asleep again, but her sleep was agitated. She was restless, probably dreaming, because all of a sudden she'd open her eyes, appear startled, and try to get up. Mom is still very strong; she can sit straight up without using her arms. Each time she did this, I soothed her and helped her to lie back again.

For the rest of the time I was there, Mom was asleep.

I can no longer speak with her by phone, although I can still call the hospital. My calls are directed to her nurse, and if the nurse is busy, to one of the aides. I receive a report—that Mom is fine, or that she's sleeping, or that she ate well. Yesterday I was told that she'd sat in her wheelchair and watched with amusement some entertainers performing. The nurses and staff are all very nice and polite to me, but they clearly are busy with other patients and tasks, and I don't want to bother them to put my mother on the phone.

On June 14, Michael sent an e-mail to Kate and Patricia. Kate forwarded a copy to me: "Doesn't qualify to go back to memory care because takes 2 people to assist to get her up and she needs close constant monitoring still."

Thus the memory-care unit's refusal to take her back made the necessary decision for us. Her belongings were to be moved out of the memory-care unit. Mom was to stay in the long-term care unit in the hospital permanently. She would no longer receive rehabilitation therapy, however, due to what turned out to be her limited progress in walking alone.

Patricia answered Michael in a message he forwarded to Kate, who sent it on to me. The message read in part:

> I suggest you cancel her phone...and clear her
> room. She hasn't been there for so long, over a

month? Therefore, I'd request a deep discount since they haven't had to care for or feed her. With all the care she's getting at the hospital, should you let that "at home" policy lapse? Not necessary to have a caretaker visit her daily.

Let us face it, at this age and condition she's not going to improve. She's at the best place for her. Thank you, Agie and Stephanie, for all your time and loving care for Mother. (Stephanie is Agnes's daughter.)

On July 8, Kate called to tell me about a new text message from Michael. Mom had a low red blood cell count and had had a transfusion two weeks after her hip surgery, possibly related to blood loss during surgery since she was on a blood thinner.

Clearly, this new placement, this "long-term care unit," would be Mother's last stop on her gradual transition from Michael's home, to a senior residence center, to the memory-care unit, and now, for the first time, to the care of professionals—trained nurses around the clock. This time it was assumed that my mother probably would never walk alone again, just as the hospice nurse had predicted two years ago, before Mom had eye surgery. "Due to losing too much core strength and having her knees bent for so long in a wheelchair," she'd said. Mother's physical state of health has been declining during her seven years of residential care. She now has been diagnosed with the following conditions among those that researchers have found associated with dementia: high blood pressure, hypothyroidism, depression, and cataracts.

Given Mother's age of ninety-three as I write this, I still believe that for a long time her stage of Alzheimer's disease was moderate.[21] Why do I think this? For one thing, advanced age is associated with an initially somewhat less severe dementia marked by fewer plaques and proportionately fewer neurofibrillary tangles. Her symptoms in the first stage when she lived in the residential-care home were primarily impaired memory (especially for recent events), repetition, and disorientation. It wasn't until after she moved to the memory-care unit that her cognitive and visual problems became worse, and she gradually lost the ability to perform the basic activities of everyday care for herself.

In terms of a prognosis, those with mild to moderate Alzheimer's conditions (e.g., problems speaking or understanding speech and performing basic Activities of Daily Living) usually live two to ten more years beyond diagnosis, although again, the rate of decline varies from person to person. If Mom's Alzheimer's had been severe when she was first diagnosed with it almost six years ago, she probably wouldn't have been able to recognize family members and likely wouldn't have been able to speak or walk as long as she has—her life span after diagnosis would've been between one and five years.

My mother retains the ability to recognize me and remember my name, and she has had very lucid moments of insight in the past three months, as in one of our last phone conversations. Her strength and resilience have astounded me while she's endured various hospitalizations, periods of hospice care, frightening months of blindness, and hip surgery.

Almost certainly she'll never go outdoors again to smell the fresh air, or feel the warmth of the sun or a cool breeze on her face, or see the flowers, the stars, or any other gifts of nature that she so loved.

As the summer wore on, Mother's condition quickly declined, both physically and mentally. By mid-August when I called, her nurse told me that Mom no longer was speaking but could respond to some verbal commands. In advanced AD, most of the cortex is seriously damaged. The brain shrinks dramatically due to widespread cell death. Individuals lose their ability to communicate, to recognize family and loved ones, and to care for themselves. For some time now the staff had been feeding her. She was either in a wheelchair or in bed, never on her feet anymore. The nurses continued to take care of the bone infections on her feet that she'd had when she entered the hospital the end of May.

A few days after my call with the nurse, a letter from Michael, sent to Kate and then on to me, confirmed what the nurse had said about Mom's feet not healing. Michael thought that the cause was poor circulation. He indicated that he was going to request less sedation. When I called the nurse, I asked if that meant Mom would be getting fewer tranquilizers, which I took Michael's letter to mean. The nurse said, "Not really tranquilizers...the doctor is backing off on psychotropic drugs." I assumed that she meant the psychotropic drugs that are antianxiety or antidepressants and not the stronger antipsychotic agents used in the treatment of schizophrenia and mania.

Now I'm planning to visit her again. Will she recognize me, be able to speak to me? Perhaps not, but even so, I want to be with her, to hug her and give her one more kiss. I'm not ready to lose her, yet I hate to see the emptiness that she's become. In my last photo of her, she's lying asleep, fully clothed on top of her bed, and I'm sitting on the chair at her side, leaning over her with my arm encircling her head as if I'm trying to protect her from something approaching. Should that be my last image, or will I see her one last time? Will she be able to hear and understand me? I hope so. Hearing is usually the last sense to go.

I went back. This time Ed went with me, and we stayed for several days to be sure we could spend enough of her waking hours with her. During those days I went into and out of the hospital's long-term care unit seven different times to visit with her, and Mom was awake and responsive about half of those occasions.

She still recognized me, but not Ed, whom she had not seen for a year or so. She looked very different since I'd last seen her three months earlier. The beautician at the hospital had cut her hair and given her a permanent; now soft, fluffy white curls framed her face.

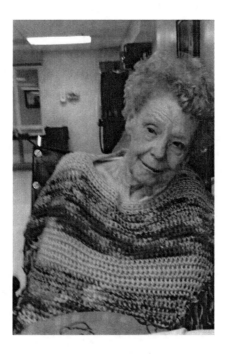

The first night we were there we sat with her and about sixteen other patients in the dining room. Only three were men, but these numbers varied as some patients apparently ate their meals in their rooms at times. Almost all of the patients in the dining room, like my mother, were sitting in wheelchairs.

She allowed me to feed her during her mealtimes, but she can and does feed herself some foods. On two different occasions she picked up sandwiches and ate them by herself; she even tried to pick up her bowls of soup, but I quickly helped her so they wouldn't spill. She also needed help not to spill her drinks, but she finished with a straw both the juice and her favorite drink, chocolate Boost, at each meal.

Her hands moved constantly as she continued her repetitive routine of counting (now only to five, not twenty) then clapping. The next day I asked the aides if there were some things we could give her so that she'd have something to do with her hands; Mom had always been busy, and there wasn't much besides her hands that she could move now, confined to the chair or the bed as she was. One of the aides found some blocks and puzzles, but stacking the colored blocks interested Mom only briefly. Instead, at the table where she sat during the day, she found a piece of colored newsprint and wrapped the blocks in it. She liked to hold this in her lap, much as she used to hold her silverware wrapped in a napkin, and her hands stopped fluttering about so much.

She still had three terrible sores on her feet, the bone infections that her doctor (not my brother) was monitoring, and I watched a nurse change the dressings on them the day after the doctor had done a debridement to remove the dead tissue and skin. I wonder how much pain she can feel; the nurse said the doctor had given her something to numb her feet before the procedure. In spite of what the nurse had told me previously over the telephone, Mom still speaks. She loudly asked the nurse what she was doing and demanded that she stop, but then she sat through the procedure without moving. Besides the medicine for her feet, she was receiving drops for glaucoma in both of her eyes twice a day. Also, she was on a blood thinner.

Conversation with her was difficult. What do you talk about with someone in her position—small talk about your own life? When I mentioned my children, she showed little recognition and asked no questions about them, although she raised her eyebrows when I told her how old they are now. Showing her pictures is pointless; her vision isn't good enough to see them, and she doesn't remember any of my twelve grandchildren. We did have a brief conversation the first night:

Me: "Do you like the people here?"
Mom: "Some of them."
Me: "Do you like it better here than where you were before?"
Mom: "No."
Me: "What did you like there?"
Mom: "More activity."

I don't know if she was referring to the fact that she was more active before or that more activity took place around her then. Certainly at the memory-care unit I never heard anyone speak like the woman who sat at the table with Mom the second evening I fed her. This lady wanted to give the aide her reading glasses, as a gift. The aide protested, saying that the woman would need them the next day so she'd just put them on the nightstand for her.

"I won't need them," was the reply. "I'm going to die tonight."

"I hate it when they say that," the aide told me.

The nurses told me that Mom is awake much of the night and that's one reason she sleeps so much during the day. I read that when melatonin levels drop in the pineal gland, darkness is no longer the cue for sleep, and in this later phase, sleeping is the norm. With so much cell damage, the patient can't stay awake. When she's in bed, they turn her from side to side every two hours around the clock to prevent bedsores. When she sits in her wheelchair, she's slouched to one side with her neck in that uncomfortable crooked position one assumes while trying to sleep on an airplane. She can no longer hold her head up for any length of time. I kept trying to place a pillow on her shoulder to support her neck and prevent it from aching, but none would stay in place. The pillow actually seemed to annoy Mom more than any neck pain she could possibly have.

*Does she dream?* I wonder. Is it the "sleep that knits up the raveled sleave [sic] of care, the death of each day's life" as Shakespeare wrote in *Macbeth*? Does she even have any cares now? For all appearances, she seems to live in a world that has shrunk to immediate sensations, a world without identity and a sleep without dreams. In her day-to-day existence, she:

- sees no familiar faces,
- is unable to read books or papers,
- is unable to watch television or movies,
- has little ability to speak,
- has lost most of her senses of taste and smell,
- is unable to walk or control any of her bodily functions, and
- has no memory.

✳✳✳

What must it be like to live with no memory of the past and no anticipation of the future? In meditation, one seeks to "be here now," to be present in the moment, the only time that actually exists, even if it is ephemeral. But the mind wanders. It refuses to stay quiet. It wants to reexamine the past and rehearse the future. We are those past memories that define us—what we've experienced, whom we love, where we've been, even what we've lost. We are those future plans and expectations that will shape us—what we look forward to next, what we desire, our hopes and ideas and dreams. When all of this disappears, when the three-pound organ that is the brain stops working, who are we? How and where will the mind wander without the brain to carry out its functions? Does a time come when we can no longer be aware that our brain isn't functioning correctly, when we don't know that we can't remember?

We have physical evidence of the brain, but the concept of mind is much more difficult to comprehend. By any definition, the mind is nonmaterial, yet it works with the brain. Is it consciousness, awareness, the overall personality, our attitudes and beliefs? Or is it something perhaps far greater, such as the human spirit or soul? Mind, or consciousness, is a timeless mystery. It's our very sense of self, the most essential part of us, yet we don't know what it is, where it comes from, or how it arises.

Hippocrates in the fifth century BC said, "To consciousness the brain is messenger," and the relationship between the two has been debated at least ever since.

The early twentieth-century psychologist William James called the mind/brain issue "the ultimate of ultimate problems." He said, "It is that our normal waking consciousness, the rational consciousness, as we call it, is but one special type of consciousness, whilst all about it, parted from it by the filmiest of screens, there lie potential forms of consciousness entirely different."[22] James believed that the mind, the "I," is the knower, the stream of consciousness, and that the "me" is the empirical self, the content.

For philosophers, the problem is referred to as dualism versus monism. Descartes—the "cogito, ergo sum" (I think, therefore I am) philosopher—Plato, Carl Jung, and others were all dualists like James and believed that the mind observes itself projecting thoughts. Kant thought there has to be some process that takes individual processing and connects it together into a unified experience. Hobbes, on the other hand, was one philosopher who believed in monism, that mental activity is explained by physical events.

In science, the same debate, now called brain/mind, is spoken of as "reductionism" and "antireductionism." Reductionism, comparable to monism, has been the modern favorite, equating brain and mind on the principle that they are inseparable. It, too, has a long history; Galen in the second century said, "Do not consult the gods to discover the directing soul, but consult an anatomist." Yet if dualists have a problem in pointing to a locale for an executive mind, reductionists also have the same problem in describing an executive brain.

A famous experiment in 1983 by Benjamin Libet, a neurophysiologist at UCSF, demonstrated that the conscious mind doesn't completely control and direct what happens in the brain. Subjects who were wired with electrodes to measure brain activity were seated where they could see a rapidly rotating clock hand and told to flex their fingers at a certain point. Libet found that the brain's neurons were firing before the conscious mind decided to give the command to flex the finger. He explained that another mechanism in the brain delayed the sensation of the finger moving so that the conscious mind believes it has controlled the action.[23] (As an aside, "The brain made me do it," would lend an interesting dimension to the subject of free will or to courtroom defenses of a "trigger happy" felon.)

According to Dr. Erik Kandel, recipient of a Nobel Prize in Physiology or Medicine for his work on memory, the new science of mind is "based on the principle that our mind and our brain are inseparable. The brain is a complex biological organ possessing immense computational capability...our mind is a set of operations carried out by our brain. The same principle of unity applies to mental disorders."[24]

Perhaps we never really do forget anything, and memories continue to exist, with or without our willing them. Cases exist of individuals who can remember everything they ever knew or experienced, down to the date and time when an event occurred. Others with post-traumatic stress disorder are troubled with memories of events they try to forget but cannot. Still others recount supposedly forgotten events with total recall under hypnosis. Finally, some individuals retain memories they can't express because of the physical limitations of the brain when neuronal connections and communication between brain regions become broken. I'm reminded of two real-life examples.

In the book and the movie *The Diving Bell and the Butterfly*,[25] the French journalist Jean-Dominique Bauby awoke twenty days after a stroke to his brain stem made him a victim of "locked-in syndrome." At the time, Bauby was forty-four years old and the editor-in-chief of the magazine *Elle*. The stroke left him mentally aware and active, but physically unable to move any part of his body except for his left eyelid, which he used to dictate his story. In his case, the mind/brain remained active, but without the connection to the body.

In the film *Awakenings*,[26] based on the non-fiction book of the same title by Dr. Oliver Sacks, hospitalized patients who had suffered from encephalitis decades earlier in the epidemic of 1917–1928 appeared to be catatonic for years until they were treated with L-Dopa, a drug that affects neurons in the basal ganglia and midbrain. For a very brief time, the patients were awakened and seemed apparently normal—active, emotional, and verbal again. But the result was short lived, and the catatonia returned. Yet even though in this example the brain had been unresponsive for years, the mind had retained abilities not experienced since childhood in most cases.

And so the question of mind/brain, or brain/mind, has long been one of the more puzzling questions in philosophy and science. For someone like my mother with Alzheimer's, does she still have her sense of self even though she's incapable of expressing it? Would it be better to keep one's mind even though the brain scarcely functions, or to let it go along with the detritus of the brain? Unfortunately, one has no choice. Like Bauby and the encephalitis patients, Alzheimer's victims are, in a sense, locked in.

✳✳✳

On one of my calls in January 2014, Mother's nurse informed me that she's much more alert and responsive than she'd been when she slept through so much of my last visit. Perhaps she's rallying once again, less than two months before her birthday. Or maybe her medications have been reduced now that one foot is healed and the other one is improving. Ed and I are making plans to visit her again soon. I'll continue to do so as long as she lives.

On Mother's birthday, March 2, 2014, she was ninety-four years old. I called that day to ask the nurse to wish her happy birthday for me since I couldn't be with her. When I inquired about her health, the nurse told me that Mom was becoming more alert and talkative yet again as she was on fewer medications now, except the one for the bone infection that remained in one foot. She was also feeding herself now unless she was tired. I'm eager to visit her again soon, this wonderful, strong lady who still is "not going gently."

Patients may live twenty years with Alzheimer's disease, and the last and most severe stage may last for six or more years. In stage seven, they have an apparent loss of reasoning capacity and a complete dependence on others for their care; they can no longer walk or even feed themselves. The loss of abilities in Alzheimer's reverses almost exactly the stages of development moving from infancy to adulthood: the hippocampus and frontal lobe are the last parts of the brain to develop in childhood and the first to be lost with

AD, and the toddler stages of learning self-care and continence are next to the last to leave before the Alzheimer's patient is as totally dependent as a newborn again, much like Shakespeare wrote in "Seven Ages of Man" (*As You Like It*):

> ...last scene of all,
> That ends this strange eventful history,
> Is second childishness and mere oblivion,
> Sans teeth, sans eyes, sans taste, sans everything.

Alzheimer's patients become vulnerable to infections and other diseases. Eventually, the motor system deteriorates: the swallowing reflex is gone, the lungs don't breathe, the heart doesn't beat. For several years AD had been called the sixth leading cause of death in the United States and the fifth leading cause of death for those over sixty-five years of age. In March 2014, however, Alzheimer's became recognized as the *third* leading cause of death in the United States; previously it had been underreported because factors like heart disease or stroke are more likely to appear on death certificates, or Alzheimer's disease is disguised as pneumonia.[27] Dementia cuts five to ten years off an average life span. Two-thirds of AD patients will die in nursing homes or hospitals, lingering, languishing, and left alone.

Mother has moved beyond our reach. We can do nothing for her. My siblings and I have tried to help, each in our own way and according to our individual levels of concern, ability, interest, and resources. But we were stretched over distances too far apart both physically and emotionally, and our lines of communication had frayed and broken. Mom's heart would have been broken, too, if she'd been aware of our conflicts. Worst of all, even with visits by Michael and Agnes who live near her and less frequent visits from my sisters and me, over the years she gradually lost all continuity of contact with her family. With her lack of responsiveness now, there's a temptation to abandon her, but I'll continue to make periodic visits.

I remain convinced that if we somehow could have found a way to keep her living with some help in one of our homes as long as possible, she could have lived with joy and happiness for a much longer time before going into residential care, if such care were ever needed. Instead, she's spent almost eight long years living among strangers in one kind of institution or another.

We gave her over to the care of strangers, yes, but they're almost all good and kind people, willing to do the things we could not—or truthfully, would not—do, things she did for all of us: change diapers, shower and help dress her, make sure she's fed and has her medications, and provide every other type of daily assistance, even entertain her.

In spite of the care, these facilities have sometimes been called "warehouses for the elderly." They're caring places for the most part, but impersonal in that all of the patients are treated alike in what is called the "institutional model"; that is, patients are defined by their disease and are often sedated so they can be more easily controlled, sometimes even with powerful psychotropic drugs that are meant for serious mental illnesses. Meanwhile, we leave our family in what has been named "God's waiting room" until each number is called, death by degrees, losing our loved ones a step at a time.

At some point Mother will be entering the final stage of severe Alzheimer's disease we've dreaded for so long. Age did not cause her worst changes. Alzheimer's did. How long the period of wasting has been, how much of her life has been robbed from her and from us. Seeing these changes in her has been like watching a slow-motion tragedy, the process of dying eating away at her mind and body until all that's left is an empty shell. She's both here and not here. Strangely I have the image of the Cheshire Cat in *Alice in Wonderland*, gradually dissolving until all that remained was the grin. Does death grin at us and mock us? I always believed death was as described, "grim."

Does Mom have any sense left of what her life used to be like, any remnant of her past identity that she can cling to? Does she think this is the way she's always been? Is she aware that she's dying? Her memory is gone, her speech is mostly silenced, but does she still feel emotions? Is she afraid, or is she in that state of "no fear," the "matter of fact lady," as her visiting angel once described her? Is she peaceful? Will her death be a relief? Or is she silently panicked, searching to find some meaning in the chaos?

I'd like to think that she's living in the eternal now, beyond the anguish of grief or guilt, sheltered from the anxiety of fears and the pull of desires. Descartes said, "I think, therefore I am." But in Buddhist philosophy, the highest pinnacle of meditation is to be beyond thought. Nirvana is a state without ego or the sense of self; it's a calm and peaceful state. Perhaps her mind is being scrubbed clean and memories erased for a spotless entry into the afterlife. Instead of a body without a working brain, perhaps she has been reduced to a soul who will be freed at last with death.

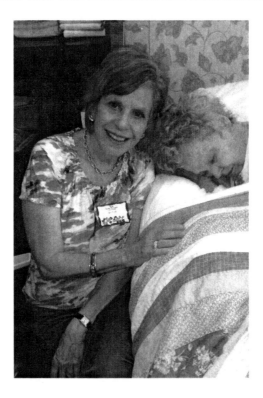

I'm haunted by the thought that my mother will likely die alone in long-term care, with no one from her family by her bedside. I'm also aware that she may no longer realize her solitude or even care.

# PART TWO:

## NEW DIRECTIONS

# CHAPTER SEVEN: A LATENT GENE

## Risk, Early Prevention, and Planning

Several months before I decided to expand my first chapter *Lost* from a short story into a book length memoir of my mother and study of Alzheimer's disease, I saw a notice in the *San Francisco Chronicle* that interested me very much. The Memory and Aging Center at UCSF was seeking volunteers for a longitudinal research study of fifteen hundred subjects, both healthy individuals and those with dementia, to explore and identify early markers of degenerative brain disease. Not only was I interested in the topic for personal reasons, as a psychologist I appreciated the value of research projects and the critical need for more volunteers if knowledge is to advance. I submitted my name as a subject. And then I forgot about it.

Meanwhile, I continued doing my own research in order to add more recent scientific information to my mother's story of cognitive decline. During this process I thought—or perhaps I was really only hoping—that I was immune from following Mother's path. After all, I had a postgraduate education, and numerous sources suggest that the more education one has, the more "cognitive reserve" is accumulated.

Cognitive reserve refers to the way the brain can continue to operate effectively in spite of sustaining some damage or disruption in function. We build cognitive reserve by the ways we use our brains, especially by keeping the brain active and mentally stimulated. More formal education is one way; being bilingual or multilingual is another, but for many of us those opportunities passed with our school years. Yet if we want to save our brain from degenerative decline, we have to find activities that will nurture it with attention every day. Social interactions, games, and leisure activities are enjoyable and entertaining, but more important is for the brain to become deeply engaged with a challenging and novel activity, preferably one that gives a sense of purpose. The additional neuron connections thus formed provide the brain with plasticity and alternate routes to compensate for any damaged areas, keeping it adaptable and flexible, and possibly decreasing the risk of dementia up to 47 percent, according to the Alzheimer's Association. In my case, I took on a new project and area of learning—this book.

I never did succumb to the medical students' disease of thinking that the symptoms I was studying were my own symptoms. Besides, I certainly knew that Alzheimer's disease isn't contagious, although it can be *genetic* in approximately 5 percent of cases, caused by a defective or mutant gene that results in early-onset AD between the ages of thirty and sixty. On the other hand, a *genetic predisposition* doesn't necessarily result in Alzheimer's unless other risk factors are also present. I knew that AD is more prevalent among females and that, according to the Alzheimer's Association, women in their sixties are about twice as likely to develop AD over the remainder of their lives as they are to develop breast cancer.[28] Yet somehow I'd managed to read over the words "APOE e4 gene" without registering their importance to me.

Several months later, as I was working on what I thought would be the last chapter in *Not Going Gently* I received a call from one of the research coordinators at UCSF. She thanked me for my interest in the aging and memory study, asked me a number of questions, and answered my queries about what my participation would involve. After telling me I'd be accepted as a healthy volunteer, she explained that there would be 750 participants and 750 study partners who also would be interviewed. She requested the name of a family member or friend who could be my partner and give a report when asked about my behavior. I volunteered my husband, Ed.

My first appointment, scheduled for the following month, was a three-hour visit beginning at noon. Included would be cognitive testing, a blood draw, and a neurological exam, all to take place at the UCSF Mission Bay campus. I'd never been there before and was surprised at the size of the campus and the number of buildings and people, but on the appointed day I found the Neurosciences Center and considered that I must have passed the first test.

The building was several stories high, very contemporary and stark, and quite sterile-looking inside. I had to sign in and wait a few minutes in an almost-empty, cavernous lobby until a research assistant I'll call Anna came for me and brought me behind locked doors. We entered a series of long hallways lined with doors closed to what I presumed were offices as well as examining rooms. Hospitals have seemed friendlier than this building did. I gave her the questionnaire I'd been asked to complete before the appointment, primarily my own evaluation of my present emotional state and cognitive ability.

We entered one of the examining rooms that held a small table, three chairs, and an examining table. Just as in the corridors, nothing in the room was warm or inviting to encourage relaxation or an opening conversation. Anna and I sat across from each other at the small table, and she introduced me to a male associate who also entered the room. Anna began by asking me the simplest questions, such as did I know where I was, what city, what county, what date this was, and so on. Once she assessed my ability to answer correctly, she gave me a number of consent forms to read, initial, and sign. The male associate in the room was probably present as a witness, but he also explained his primary role. He was there to discuss the autopsy program and encourage me to sign the consent forms to donate my brain and spinal cord for research. I took the forms from him and indicated that I'd probably sign them. Then he left.

Anna then led me to another room where a phlebotomist took a sample of my blood for serum, plasma, and genetic analysis. Possibly my cells would be grown and immortalized without my identification as a cell line for future use in scientific studies at the National Cell Repository for Alzheimer's Disease (NCRAD).

Back in the original room, the fun began, except that it wasn't fun at all. The tests started out to be easy enough but rapidly progressed in difficulty. Many of them involved listening to long lists of unrelated, mixed up words, then repeating back as many as I could remember, sometimes after an intervening list of different words. I tried to group the words into the four categories they represented (foods, furniture, means of transportation, animals) while Anna was saying them, but that mental activity seemed to interfere with my concentration on echoic or hearing impressions and to actually lessen the total number I could remember. Numbers were better; I could recall a list of nine random numbers and recite them backward when asked. There were timed tests of sixty seconds each, such as saying all the words I could that began with the letter *d*, or naming as many animals as I could, without repeating any. I was slower than I thought I'd be because I was afraid of repeating. Next, I was given drawings to look at and then, after an interval with other tests in between, asked to reproduce as much of a particular drawing as I could. I thought I did all right but knew I certainly missed some details. Another paper and pencil test didn't seem complicated, but it was timed also and I made two errors. I was tired, and since I'd been instructed not to eat before arriving due to the blood tests, I felt less alert. As I was slowing down in responding, I was becoming stressed and frustrated because of my obvious mistakes.

No longer feeling like a good student, I was very uncomfortable seeing myself in this diminished role. I knew that as we age there is a shrinking of neurons and a reduction both in the level of neurotransmitters and the blood flow to the brain, making responses slower, but I hadn't been confronted by speed tests for a long time and was surprised to see just how slow my ability to respond had become. Nevertheless, as Anna led me down the hall to where a neurologist would test my reflexes, eye movements and so on, she told me confidentially that I did fine and didn't need to worry.

But worry I did. The tests tore a large hole in my aura of confidence. Perhaps my parents' genes were a more critical factor for my cognitive health than my education level was, after all. For many years I've struggled to control high LDL cholesterol like my father had, and recently I've been bothered with osteoarthritis, just as both parents were. My eye doctor has told me that I'm beginning to get cataracts, and for a number of years I've had to use eye drops to prevent glaucoma. Might I also be starting on the path to dementia? I went back to my research and this time paid much closer attention to the APOE e4 gene.

The acronym APOE e4 stands for a protein called apolipoprotein E, a lipoprotein, considered to be beneficial when it carries the good HDL cholesterol and fats the brain needs through the bloodstream. In fact, some scientists worry that the statin drugs to lower cholesterol may be depriving the brain of needed fats even as statins help prevent cardiovascular diseases. Yet APOE e4 also appears to act at times in the formation of amyloid plaques. The gene associated with APOE is on chromosome 19, and every person inherits two of them, one from each parent. Since the gene has three different versions, called alleles, there are six possible combinations, each presenting a different risk level for developing Alzheimer's disease. Allele e2 is considered rare, but may provide some protection against Alzheimer's. Allele e3 is the most common, considered neutral or default. Allele e4 is the problem; it occurs in 20 to 30 percent of the general population, but 40 to 65 percent of all people with late-onset AD, or LOAD, have one or two copies of APOE e4.[29]

One copy of APOE e4 increases Alzheimer's risk approximately three times, with symptoms showing by age seventy-five instead of at eighty-four, the average age of symptom onset for individuals with no copies of the allele. With two copies of APOE e4, an individual has a 50 percent chance of developing Alzheimer's by age eighty, and 12 to 15 percent of these individuals may already begin showing symptoms by the age of sixty-eight.[30] Between the ages of sixty-eight and eighty-four, that difference is really significant. Also, sex should be taken into account; the APOE e4 gene has been described as having a "nastier affect" on women.

These numbers represent risk and don't predict with certainty that the presence of APOE e4 in the blood means the person will develop Alzheimer's disease. Genes are considered to be responsible for only about a third of our physical and mental health. In the longitudinal Nun Study started in 1986 of sisters from the same religious order, the autopsy of one nun who died at the age of 107 revealed one copy of the APOE e4 allele, but she had never displayed signs of dementia. I don't know if my blood test at UCSF was intended to discover, among other things, which allele combination of APOE may be present in my blood, but I suspect it was among the components being evaluated. In any case, I won't be told the result. Individuals in this study don't receive feedback. The reason is to avoid useless anxiety, since no medical management (i.e., treatment) exists.

Anxiety may be a useless emotion; nonetheless, I felt its presence. Suddenly every word or name I forgot, every mental blank, became an ominous sign. I wish I could remember how old my mother was when her symptoms began, but I was living in northern California by then and only seeing her periodically throughout the year. At those times, as I said earlier, I thought she repeated herself and asked others to repeat conversations because she wasn't paying close enough attention. As nearly as I can recall, however, I believe that she may have been showing early symptoms by the time she was seventy-three, my age now. So I was making certain that I paid extra attention to what was being said around me, and I mentally congratulated myself whenever I remembered something quickly. Even if I thought a conversation was irrelevant to me and not worth remembering, I focused on it anyway. And I did focus!

Consulting my notes again, I reread a report from Gary Small, MD, director of the UCLA Longevity Center on Aging, who says, "The idea that Alzheimer's is entirely genetic and unpreventable is perhaps the greatest misconception about the disease. Researchers now know that Alzheimer's, like heart disease and cancer, develops over decades, and can be influenced by lifestyle factors, including cholesterol, blood pressure, obesity, depression, education, nutrition, sleep, and mental, physical, and social activity."[31]

In fact, the very same risk factors that contribute to cardiovascular disease—unhealthy weight, Type 2 diabetes, high blood pressure, smoking, lack of exercise, and high LDL / low HDL cholesterol—contribute to dementia as well. According to Dr. Small, being overweight in middle age doubles the risk of dementia, and obesity raises the risk by four times.[32] Diabetes and high blood pressure both increase brain shrinkage, and high blood pressure causes the myelin sheath to decay. Heart health is strongly associated with brain health.

Dr. Small and many others state the current opinion: that prevention is today's only available cure. Right here and now we can prevent Alzheimer's. Up to half of the risk for Alzheimer's disease is potentially under our control.

We are living in a period of historical change with the opportunity to do something that our ancestors never imagined. For earlier generations like my grandparents', dementia wasn't a worry; the life span was shorter, and most people didn't face the increased risk that old age brings. For my father, heart problems had always been a primary concern, and I think he was actually surprised at the mental decline that overtook him near the end of his life. His age group had never considered a need for prevention. My mother has lived much longer with her dementia, yet unfortunately she was in the cohort group treated with drugs that were too little, too late to help. But for those of us who are seniors now, we can take advantage of numerous studies and reports that for the first time ever are daring to say we can stave off dementia. (For those who are still baby boomers, the potential exists to eliminate AD in their future.)

I began making what other changes I could initiate to fight back. Of the key proactive strategies for prevention—exercise, nutrition, meaningful social connections, and mental stimulation—only the first one listed, exercise, wasn't covered in my mother's story. Yes, my mother walked a lot, but for her and others who were wanderers or who walked to reduce agitation, exercise was probably like the medications they were given—too little, too late.

But now we're speaking of exercise, especially walking, to prevent Alzheimer's, and it's being mentioned most frequently as the "best thing you can do for your brain." The evidence that physical activity is beneficial to the brain comes from a number of large epidemiological studies and a variety of medical experts. In spite of this, a reported 60 percent of Americans aren't regularly physically active, and 25 percent don't exercise at all.[33]

"If we had a pill that could do what exercise does, its sales would put Viagra's to shame," says Laura L. Carstensen, director of the Stanford Center on Longevity and author of *A Long Bright Future*. "The latest research shows that cognitive decline is not inevitable. Yes, brain volume shrinks slightly. But the brain continues to make new neurons and fine-tune neural connections as long as we live."[34]

Kirk Erickson, associate professor of psychology at the University of Pittsburgh, agrees that exercise is good for the brain. "We see changes in brain regions that typically show decline and deterioration later in life. The brain shrinks, unfortunately, as we get older. But research has proven that the brain remains highly modifiable into late adulthood. And exercise is one way to modify it," he says. Erickson should know. He was one of the key authors in a study of dementia-free people sixty to seventy-nine years old who walked briskly three times a week. After the six-month program, the increase in the size of the hippocampus and the levels of BDNF [brain-derived neuropathic factor] were comparable to those found in people almost two years younger. "This was the first time that we were able to demonstrate that you can actually increase the size of the hippocampus," Erickson says.[35]

How does exercise change the brain? By boosting the flow of blood to the brain, exercise releases more of the memory protein called BDNF. This protein is a growth factor that stimulates the formation of new neurons in the hippocampus, repairs cell damage, and strengthens synapses. By increasing the size of the hippocampus, BDNF helps mediate the damage or shrinkage caused by depression and/or dementia. BDNF possibly also protects against beta-amyloid toxicity and preserves cognition in older adults.

And exercise helps improve HDL levels, the form of cholesterol critical for the brain to use. John Medina, an affiliate professor of bioengineering at the University of Washington School of Medicine and author of *Brain Rules*, suggests that aerobic exercise can jump-start the process. He says, "It also slashes your lifetime risk of Alzheimer's in half and your risk of general dementia by 60 percent."[36]

Experts agree that exercise can begin at any age. Erickson says that his study "was as if we'd rolled back the clock. It proves that exercising even in late adulthood, even if you've not been active before, isn't futile. People need to know that dementia isn't inevitable."

People like me will also be glad to know that the American Heart Association's recommendation for moderate exercise for thirty minutes at least five days a week brought the highest benefit to those individuals who have the greatest risk for late-onset Alzheimer's disease, the people with APOE e4. According to the report first published in 2012, "those who met or exceeded AHA guidelines reduced their brain amyloid deposits to levels similar to those seen in people who didn't have the APOE e4 gene."[37]

One further benefit of exercise is that, like meditation, it can reduce the stress hormone cortisol that affects depression and anxiety and can damage the brain's white matter pathways, interfering with communication between regions. I take a yoga class at least once a week, and adding meditation to my daily routine gave me the additional benefit described in a UCLA study showing that meditation increases folding in the cerebral cortex that helps in processing information.[38]

Earlier (in Chapter Three) I discussed the Mediterranean diet and listed important supplements, especially the B Vitamins, Vitamin $D_3$, glutathione, EFAs, and Alpha lipoic acid. I continue to take those, but now with further research I have made some changes to update my list for nutrition:

- I added raw nuts and seeds to my diet, continued to eat wild salmon once or twice a week, and continued to put olive oil on my daily salads in order to increase my level of EFAs, especially omega-3 (DHA), which some studies show may help to reduce beta-amyloid plaques.[39]

- I also eliminated most animal protein from my diet. I'd long ago given up eating any meat other than poultry. But now I almost completely stopped eating it as well, along with many dairy products, in an attempt to reduce my LDL cholesterol level.

- Instead of drinking white wine, I switched to having red wine for its antioxidant components, usually having one glass a day at dinnertime. (One study showed that moderate drinking of one to six alcoholic beverages a week, usually of wine, could *slow* the progression from mild cognitive impairment to more serious dementia by 85 percent compared to not drinking.[40] Another study reported that mild to moderate drinking could *reduce the risk* of developing dementia by 54 percent compared to not drinking.[41] Scientists believe that moderate alcohol consumption improves the blood flow to the brain and may help prevent small strokes. However, drinking alcohol has its risks, and those who don't drink are warned not to start; binge drinking in midlife more than triples the risk of developing dementia in later life.)[42]

• Besides consuming more glasses of pure water, my other beverages include coffee, green tea, and an occasional cup of cocoa. A new Harvard University study indicates drinking two cups of cocoa a day for thirty days significantly improved memory in older adults.[43] The same amount, about 500 grams, of strong coffee a day in midlife cut Alzheimer's risk 65 percent in late life in a large European study. Caffeine may be the key component in both of these beverages. And the Alzheimer's Association reports that only a cup of black or green tea a week cut rates of cognitive decline in older people by 37 percent, probably due to its antioxidants.

• I easily added the recommended ounce or so of dark chocolate a day. Dark chocolate with a cocoa content of at least 70 percent is loaded with flavonols, the same beneficial compounds found in berries, red wine, and tea. Besides improving blood flow to the brain, some studies still in an early phase suggest flavonol compounds may also promote neurogenesis (development of new neurons) as well as improve the connections between neurons. At the very least, those who consumed the most chocolate reported feeling calmer and more content.

• Although dark chocolate is beneficial in small amounts, sugar apparently is not. In one study of 141 individuals with an average age of 63.1, higher glucose levels had a negative effect on cognition and memory, apparently due to reduced hippocampus microstructure.[44]

• I occasionally took NSAIDs like ibuprofen (e.g., Advil) and naproxen (e.g., Aleve) for my osteoarthritis. If my mother had taken these more often for her rheumatoid arthritis, their affect of reducing inflammation in the brain might have made her less likely to develop Alzheimer's disease— before the disease was already present and if there had been no family history of it before her. (Long-term use of NSAIDs, however, can lead to other side effects and isn't recommended.)[45]

I should also mention that I'm avoiding the known substances that possibly accelerate dementia:

- Valium (use Xanax or Ativan for anxiety instead)
- Benadryl, Sominex, and others that contain diphenhydramine, an anticholinergic that counteracts transmitters such as acetylcholine, important for the brain (previously mentioned in Chapter Four)
- Hypothyroid drugs, Prednisone, and corticosteroids (they can impair memory and cause confusion and irritability)
- Nicotine (narrows blood vessels in the brain)
- Alcohol (in excess; AMA says more than fourteen drinks a week for males and seven drinks a week for females increase risk.)

Once I create and embark on a plan of action and do all I can to solve a problem, I can generally stop worrying about it. Following the steps above usually works fine for me in this regard—during the daytime. Nights, however, are sometimes a different matter. Normally I sleep well for seven or eight hours throughout the night, and that's good. The brain's glial cells form new neuronal connections, prune old ones, and consolidate new learning during sleep, as well as clear out some of the beta-amyloid and tau cells.

But on those occasions when I half awaken from a dream, I have a hard time going back to sleep if I allow any thoughts to begin. A few nights after my interview at UCSF I awoke and for some reason couldn't think of the name of a prominent politician who once led a march for social justice across the Golden Gate Bridge. Ed and I had participated in that walk as we had in some other marches for peace, but I had no idea why this person should pop into my head except that it was the middle of the night when strange thoughts can and do occur. Trying to recover his name was as impossible as trying to recall a dream when what the noted psychologist William James called "the filmiest of screens" descends between the dreaming and waking states and blocks the way back to the dream, no matter how hard one may try to penetrate the screen. Of course, possibly at such times I was still experiencing half awake alpha brain waves and wasn't fully awake in beta waves. Once I did worry myself into an alert state, I eventually remembered the name. On such occasions when the sought-after word or answer finally does pop into the mind, it brings a resulting sense of immediate release. A neuron firing across a synapse has finally met the right partner. A connection has been made. Yes!

Still, if my memory were to remain frozen in the middle of the night, I could lie in bed for hours with increasing nighttime fears that I was already experiencing cognitive impairment because my mind was a blank, believing that I was experiencing some stage of dementia and looking into the abyss of Alzheimer's disease, its dark matter swallowing and extinguishing my mind's inner lights one by one. On those occasions, the horror of outliving my mind was the worst thing I could imagine. I dreaded losing my memory and my sense of self. I abhorred the very idea of being helpless and the shame of becoming a physical and financial burden to my children. Really, there are no words to adequately describe my feelings; none are strong enough. Once when I told Ed the next day about my nocturnal terror, he was teasingly reassuring. "Your mother was several years older than you are now when she started having problems," he told me. "You have some time left."

Fortunately, as some of my "time left" went by and my reaction to the tests at UCSF faded, I had no more nighttime fears about losing my memory. Granted, my recall was slower than when I was younger, but I held to my belief that as we grow older, even normal brains take longer to make the connections between neurons. In fact, recent data-mining analyses are questioning whether the reason for slower recall is age, or rather the greater amount and type of information in the brain. As an article in *The New York Times* concluded, "It's not that you're slow. It's that you know so much."[46]

My fears, although temporary, did confirm for me the mixture of feelings and reactions that many report when adjusting to a diagnosis of AD: acute grief and mourning at the thought of losing their identity and anxiety about the future. Some may also feel anger, denial, or even embarrassment. Alzheimer's is an incurable disease, and the individual may not want to know the diagnosis, or the family may want to spare the patient that knowledge. As clinicians are now trying to diagnose it in the early stages, however, informed patients will have the time and the capacity to make important decisions about their futures.

In my own "time left," what can I do individually to prepare for a better experience than my mother had? The lessons I learned from my mother's experience are the last gift she gave to me. I want to follow her example and "not go gently," but instead of relying on others' decisions, I want to make my own careful plans now while I still can, in case I'm unable to do so at some point.[47] For example, if I'm unable to care for myself, I don't want to be kept alive artificially or continue to receive treatments for illness, in spite of modern medicine's propensity for doing every kind of procedure to prolong life over all other considerations and at all costs (including financial).

The most important thing I can do differently than my parents is to have a discussion with our five adult offspring, all of them present at the same time, so they can each understand my wishes, ask questions, and agree to share their efforts in whatever care I'd need. I'd like them to discuss openly who's willing to take responsibility for handling financial decisions and making monetary and other records available for the others to see. Ed and I have a family trust and an executor of our estate, but I'd need one of the children to have my power of attorney if I outlive Ed.

To help them when that time comes, I plan to put together a folder containing vital personal information they can access, such as the following:[48]

- My durable power of attorney
- My advance directive for health-care decisions
- My doctors' names and contact information
- A list of my current medications and dosages
- A list of my drug allergies
- Passwords and records for various accounts, financial and others
- Insurance information
- The autopsy permit that I signed for the research study
- Preferences for my obituary and memorial service to relieve them from the details
- A list of persons to contact upon my death
- A will for my personal possessions, such as jewelry

In spite of my plans and good intention, however, I'm as guilty as the next person of what Ernest Becker called *Denial of Death*, his 1974 Pulitzer prize–winning book, and so far I've procrastinated. But I think if we can all discuss these issues openly and honestly we can avoid the secrecy and disagreements that my siblings and I so unfortunately had.

While it may seem very pessimistic to discuss these matters, figures show that it's realistic to be prepared. As the rates are on the rise and not declining, many more people will die from Alzheimer's disease in the future. According to the Alzheimer's Association, 61 percent of the seventy-year-olds with AD are expected to die within a decade compared to 30 percent of that same age group without AD, and one in every three seniors dies with AD or some other dementia.

Many people my age ask two questions when they hear that someone has died: How old was she or he? And what was the cause of death? These are the two final unknowns. Now I have another unanswered question to add: Do I have the APOE e4 gene combination that *may* lead to Alzheimer's disease? I'm living with the doubt now, but then, are we not all, in one manner or another, living with doubts?

In the past few years, Ed and I have lost some very good friends. Faced with questions of our own mortality, I wrote this poem, *Speaking of Death*:

We're speaking of death now, my husband and I.
We're of an age when many of our friends are dying,
Some, slowly and painfully,
Others, shockingly, suddenly.

We need to make plans.
We talk about what the surviving one would do.

Of all the questions we have asked of Life,
These are the last few unknowns that remain to us:
Where would just one of us live?
Is it better to sell our house? Buy a condo?
Live alone or go to a retirement home?
Is there enough money to provide for one's future?

But these are the easier questions.
Already we have made some harder decisions.
We have bought a cemetery plot for him, and
Recognized that her ashes will be there, too.
What kind of clothes will he be buried in?
Where will the service be?
Who will give our eulogies, and who will come?

We ask no questions of Death itself,
How It will come and when,
Solitary, shrouded mysteries
To ponder deep on a sleepless night.

It will be much easier for us if we die together,
Victims of some car or plane crash,
United in death, spared the grieving and the loneliness
And the questions that no longer matter.

The greater part of my professional teaching career was in developmental psychology. I wanted to study the process of change in normal individuals over the life cycle as they grew and evolved physically, mentally, emotionally, and spiritually. I thought of life as being divided into stages, each stage opening up to a fuller and broader experience of enrichment. Is it not ironic that my final major study in life is just the opposite?

Yet in my personal "time left," I have strong hopes that the number of scientists working in so many different research areas will at last solve the mystery of Alzheimer's disease and, once the cause is known, be able to eradicate it. I'm looking ahead with optimism, as I'll explain next.

# CHAPTER EIGHT: LOOKING AHEAD

## Numbers, Latest Developments, and Strategies

Alzheimer's disease isn't a part of normal aging, as I continue to repeat. But are we in danger of its perhaps becoming the "new" normal as more people are living longer and are therefore exposed to prolonged risk? Thousands more are developing Alzheimer's disease each day. In 2013, a new diagnosis was made every sixty-eight seconds. Unless medical breakthroughs occur, by 2050 a new diagnosis will occur every thirty-three seconds, tripling the current number of 5.4 million Alzheimer's patients to between 11 and 16 million people with AD in the United States alone.

Worldwide figures indicate just how huge and widespread the problem is. The Alzheimer's Association estimates globally every four seconds another person is considered to have AD. Alzheimer's Disease International, at the first-ever gathering of G8 Dementia Summit leaders in 2013, estimated 44 million people around the globe suffer from dementia, up from the 35 million in 2010. By 2050 the number of cases is expected to be 135 million. The World Health Organization and the Centers for Disease Control and Prevention list similar projections. Given these figures, many are concerned that we're facing a virtual "time bomb" of an impending epidemic, an unprecedented health-care crisis, particularly in lower- and middle-income areas. A worldwide effort is seeking better ways to treat, delay, and prevent AD.

As the numbers increase, so do the costs. Harry Johns, President and CEO of the Alzheimer's Association (AA), has pointed out that the economic costs of AD rival the human devastation that it causes. The AA estimates the worldwide cost of treating dementia was 604 billion dollars in 2010 and expects it to surpass 1 trillion dollars in 2050. In the United States, the AA lists the 2014 costs of caring for people with Alzheimer's and other dementias at 214 billion dollars annually, including 150 billion dollars in costs to Medicare and Medicaid. The total US costs are projected to be 1.2 trillion dollars annually by 2050.

Lawmakers in the United States are beginning to take notice. Senator Susan Collins from Maine, the top Republican on the Senate Aging Committee, recently said in a December 2013 AARP Bulletin interview, "I firmly believe that we need to have a major investment in research into Alzheimer's disease....We're spending $200 billion a year caring for people with Alzheimer's—$142 billion of that is from Medicare and Medicaid—and yet we invest a measly $500 million in research into Alzheimer's. That makes no sense whatsoever."[49]

The five hundred million dollars invested for Alzheimer's research that Senator Collins mentioned pales in comparison to the budgeted six billion dollars for cancer, five billion dollars for heart disease, and three billion dollars for HIV/AIDS. Costs and number of deaths from other diseases have declined: between 2000 and 2010, deaths from prostate cancer declined by 8 percent; from heart disease, 16 percent; from stroke, 23 percent; and from HIV, 42 percent. Figures for Alzheimer's disease have only grown. In that same ten-year period, deaths from Alzheimer's disease increased by 68 percent.[50] As stated earlier, AD is recognized now to be the third leading cause of death from disease, previously having been underreported on death certificates.

In 2014 President Obama signed into law an unprecedented 122-million-dollar increase in the budget allocated for Alzheimer's research, education, outreach, and caregiver support, the largest funding increase ever, although still considered to be not nearly enough. But the Affordable Care Act provides help as well. An e-mail I received from California Senator Dianne Feinstein on March 14, 2014, points out that the Affordable Care Act not only allows those with a preexisting condition of early-onset Alzheimer's to purchase affordable health insurance, it also entitles Medicare beneficiaries to an assessment of cognitive function, allowing seniors the chance to detect Alzheimer's as early as possible.

A significant shift of focus from treatment to prevention is taking place. In the past, it's now recognized, treatments were unsuccessful partly because they were started too late; memory and thinking problems had begun decades before symptoms manifested. The new emphasis on prevention is aided by the fact that early detection through biomarkers has now made it possible to assess an individual's risk in the earliest phases of the disease. An international study evaluating a variety of presymptomatic markers in 128 genetically predisposed subjects detected a decrease in spinal fluid levels that precedes the formation of beta-amyloid plaques twenty-five years before the anticipated onset of symptoms.[51] Plaques later show on brain scans fifteen years before memory problems are apparent. Similar precursors of fifteen years have been detected for the presence of tau and for shrinkage of key brain structures. Prevention studies naturally target those who are known to have a genetic risk, giving great hope to me and to millions of others who may be worried about genetic predisposition or early symptoms of memory loss.

One of the largest federal grants for prevention studies so far, 33.2 million dollars, was awarded to test healthy people aged sixty to seventy-five who have two copies of APOE e4, the variant that means they're up to fourteen times more likely to get AD.[52]

Dr. Lennart Mucke, director of the Gladstone Institute at UCSF says, "One of the most underinvestigated and underexploited areas in Alzheimer's research is APOE—it's nature's clue in how to avoid the disease."[53] Like other clues, however, APOE is tricky. Although it's clearly associated with the most common form of Alzheimer's disease, LOAD, not everyone who develops Alzheimer's has the APOE e4 allele.

Teasing out the role of genes and identifying them is an essential step. Scientists will then be able to take into account how genetic factors interact with lifestyle and environmental factors. The goal, even more important than developing drugs and treatments, is to prevent and stop Alzheimer's disease. Already, recent genetic studies present exciting clues:

- A team at Columbia University Medical Center led by Nobel laureate Dr. Eric Kandel looked at a certain gene in the hippocampus that, when it stops working correctly, produces less of a key protein, named RbAp48, in older people, causing age-related memory loss. Their study in the journal *Science Translational Medicine* reported that when the RbAp48 protein is given to mice, normal memory loss can be reversed, showing that age-related memory loss is distinct from Alzheimer's disease and is treatable. "It's the best evidence so far," Dr. Kandel says.[54] Until a pill can be developed, the therapies suggested for boosting the protein include exercise (both physical and cognitive) and vitamin supplements.

- A gene mutation that leads to the buildup of the protein tau in the brain has been reversed by a group of scientists at the Gladstone Institute at UCSF. They used the patient's own skin cells, regressed them to stem-cell state, then developed those stem cells into neurons to destroy the damaging tau.[55]

- The Gladstone Institute at UCSF is also making news with the "longer-life" hormone called klotho (named for Fate in Greek mythology), encoded by a variant of the gene KL-VS. Since klotho has been known to promote longevity, researchers wondered if it could also prevent cognitive decline in aging. Unfortunately, the seven hundred subjects, aged fifty-two to eighty-five, had just as much cognitive decline over time as the nonklotho control group, but they *did* have better performance at any age because klotho seemed to improve their cognitive reserve. Further experiments with mice showed that klotho increased the protein GluN2B that strengthens synaptic connections.[56]

- A related study at Stanford and UCSF in which old mice were given blood from young ones showed that the transfusion helped the old mice perform better. One question now is whether there is more klotho in young blood in humans and in mice.[57]

- Most recently, CBS news reported that eleven new gene variants linked to Alzheimer's have been discovered in the largest genetic analysis of the disease ever undertaken, doubling the known gene variants from eleven to twenty-two. The researchers performed brain scans on 74,076 older volunteers—with and without Alzheimer's disease—from fifteen countries. While APOE e4 still has a strong impact on risk, one of the newer gene variants discovered, known as HLA-DRB5/DRB, is considered to be of special interest. It's involved in an area that controls how white blood cells interact, once again pointing to the involvement of the immune system in Alzheimer's disease, as it is in multiple sclerosis and Parkinson's.[58]

- On February 12, 2014, the Alzheimer's Association and two different Parkinson's groups (the Michael J. Fox Foundation and the W. Garfield Weston Foundation of Canada) announced their offer of joint research grants to study and compare these two degenerative diseases that together affect six million Americans, hoping to lead to earlier diagnoses and targeted treatments for both.

A number of advances in other areas of research also appear to be very promising. Among these are studies looking at the role of proteins, brain structure, or insulin in the development of AD:

- A recent article reported in *The Journal of Neuroscience* points to the involvement of a protein called C1q in the development of AD and other brain disorders. Although C1q is usually part of the natural immune response, Stanford University scientists recently discovered that C1q accumulates near the synapses at much higher levels in older tissue, both mouse and human, and can destroy the synapses if the immune response is triggered for some reason. C1q is now another potential target protein like beta-amyloid and tau. Efforts are underway to develop drugs to stop the immune reaction associated with C1q.[59]

- A different study at Stanford University looked at the role of a protein called beclin in the development of AD. Beclin works to recycle immune cells called microglia that sweep the brain of foreign invaders and destructive debris before they destroy neurons. Without enough beclin, the microglia recycling is diminished. Beclin is also considered to be an important research target for other brain diseases, such as Parkinson's.[60]

- At University of California Irvine, Matthew Blurton-Jones considers synaptic loss to be the best correlate of cognitive impairment in AD. He's using modified stem cells to deliver therapeutic protein (brain-derived neuropathic factor, or BDNF) to strengthen the synapses. Results in mice to date show improved cognition in learning tests and modified disease pathology.[61]

- Researchers at University of California Davis used magnetic resonance imaging to examine the brains of 102 normal people with an average age of seventy-three. Over a five-year period of repeated scans, about 20 percent of the subjects began to show symptoms of either MCI or AD. The differences between them and the normal subjects were changes in the fornix, an organ that carries messages to and from the hippocampus. Clues to future cognitive decline may be predicted from degeneration of the fornix.[62]

- A rather unique study is testing insulin levels in the brain after finding that people with prediabetes had low insulin levels in the brain in spite of high levels in the blood. Raising insulin levels in the brain with a nasal spray has had good results so far in people with MCI or early Alzheimer's. Insulin receptors in the brain may also affect beta-amyloid and inflammation, as well as cortisol levels that are sensitive to insulin.[63]

Earlier detection would be a key critical component to any of these studies. If Alzheimer's could be detected and diagnosed early—with the knowledge that preventive treatment would be available before any symptoms appeared—more people would be agreeable to undergo tests for early diagnosis. As yet, such a certain diagnostic tool doesn't exist, but the search is underway.

One new approach would be an accurate blood test such as the one a team at UCLA is working on. In April 2014 they compared a microarray-based blood test on forty-four subjects with Alzheimer's disease and fifty-three age-matched controls. The test was accurate for all of the AD patients but gave a false positive to three of the controls, for an overall accuracy of 95 percent. So far the test is promising, and in the future it may be useful in diagnosing AD two to three years before the start of symptoms.[64]

In terms of future treatment, a team of Stanford researchers led by Dr. Ada Poon has developed tiny implants, about the size of a grain of rice, which can be controlled wirelessly to stimulate electrical impulses deep within the body. Scientists and others hope this new field of research called bioelectronics or "electroceuticals" may someday be able to influence neurosignals to treat malfunctions in the central nervous system, including diseases like Alzheimer's, Parkinson's, and many more.[65]

Alzheimer's disease is complex. Similar to other diseases such as cardiovascular disease and diabetes, it's most likely caused by a combination of factors, including genes, environment, and lifestyle factors of education, occupation, exercise, stress, and diet. But just as the causes of other complex diseases are now known, the causes of Alzheimer's will also be known one day, and scientists will then be able to concentrate on interventions. Immunizations and antioxidants may be helpful in the future, along with cognitive training to build brain reserves as people learn to use social interactions, linguistic abilities, occupations, and leisure more effectively.

Until that time, advances in the treatment and care of patients need to continue. Recognizing that most seniors prefer to stay in their own homes, where they are surrounded by the memorabilia of their lifetimes, the *Staying Put* programs use the "takes a village" concept developed in Beacon Hill Village, Boston, to provide concierge-type assisted living at home. With the help of local volunteers, neighbors, the police for safety, and other helpers, seniors can rely on transportation, food and medicine delivery, and a variety of other services while "aging in place." Besides offering the peace of mind that comes from living at home, this approach is much more affordable financially than an assisted living residence and is so popular it's spreading to other cities as the *Village to Village Network*. Other families are learning to utilize new technology to monitor parents who wish to stay in their own homes, by remotely checking on such things as their medication intake, for example.

Senior day-care centers offer many activities for those who live at home either independently or under the care of family members. As a member of a large volunteer group formed to aid seniors, I recently visited the day-care center, established in 1978, that we help support. On any given day, approximately 60 seniors out of the 150 registered are present from eight thirty in the morning to four thirty in the afternoon to receive benefits that include exercise, vital therapies, socialization, arts and crafts, and a nutritious meal and snacks. Such centers do more than provide an outing and support for patients with conditions like Parkinson's, Alzheimer's, and dementia. They offer a much-needed, valuable day of respite for family caregivers.

The daily challenges of in-home care exact a heavy toll of physical and emotional stresses on caregivers. The Alzheimer's Association estimates that last year, 15.4 million family members or friends cared for seven out of every ten patients in differing stages of Alzheimer's or other dementias. They provided 17.5 billion hours of unpaid in-home care, valued at 216.4 billion dollars. Only 47 percent of them were able to keep their regular, paid jobs; not surprisingly, 70 percent reported their finances were strained, along with the 60 percent who rated their emotional stress as very high. Depression, reported by more than one-third, further increased caregivers' lowered immunity and susceptibility to diseases, including high blood pressure and insulin levels. Much has been written elsewhere about the need for caregivers to also receive care themselves.

For those who are unable or unwilling to accept the increasing difficulties of in-home care as the patients' needs progress, other options exist, each one providing a successively higher level of supervision and treatment. As in my mother's case, residential-care homes similar to the one where she lived for two years offer lodging, meals, and some assistance with Activities of Daily Living. Her next step was moving to a memory-care unit that added secure assisted living and extra attention; Mother spent five years in the memory-care unit. Her final stay has been in a hospital that offers long-term custodial care, including twenty-four-hour monitoring, skilled nursing, and medical assistance for patients unable to care for themselves.

In any of these options, licenses require that the facility meet basic safety requirements, including state fire regulations. The staff, selected only after careful background checks, should be specially trained and offered ongoing educational programs in handling the challenges particular to dementia care and Alzheimer's. The family should ask how medical, dental, and vision needs are met, as well as question cleanliness and safety, comfort, meals, activities, and costs. Obviously, patients shouldn't be treated as victims in a warehouse or stigmatized with labels. Care shouldn't be what has been referred to as "impersonal, intermittent, and imprecise."

Too late I learned that institutional care where patients are all treated more or less the same isn't the only option. Individualized care for the elderly already exists, although it's more difficult to find. In 1997 Thomas Kitwood, a British social psychologist, published his final book, *Dementia Reconsidered: The Person Comes First,* stressing attentive treatment with more sensitivity, based on the recognition that Alzheimer's patients are still capable of feeling a wide range of emotions, including joy. Their diagnosis shouldn't define them. His ideas have been applied primarily in Europe, but more recently in the United States, particularly at the Beatitudes Campus. A retirement center near Phoenix, Arizona, the Beatitudes Campus has been described as "an incubator for a holistic model of care." The director, Tena Alonzo, says, "When you have dementia, we can't change the way you think, but we can change the way you feel."[66]

Much can be done to improve the typical residential-care experience, including allowing for more laughter and these ideas for future care:

- Already a number of senior-care homes are adding laptops for their residents to use. Many of today's seniors aren't computer literate, however, and are having some difficulty even learning to play the games designed to improve memory. But the next age group, the baby boomers, should be able to enjoy using computers because they already know how, and they'll rely on their long-term procedural memory to continue doing so. The University of California Irvine is using computer games to stimulate new connections between neurons, building on the brain's capacity for plasticity. For those who have more capability, laptops and tablets could improve cognition and mental skills as well as levels of communication and socialization.

- Access to a telephone feature like Skype would allow some patients to have video conversations at will and help them overcome their feelings of isolation and loneliness.
- Wearable cameras such as those developed by Google could help patients with impaired memories. An article in *The Economist* from November 16, 2013, states, "Research shows that patients encouraged to regularly review their lives by looking at a photo stream stand a better chance of remembering important events or conversations. There is hope that such approaches could alleviate some symptoms of dementia and Alzheimer's disease and make coping with them easier, both for the afflicted and their carers [sic]."
- A smartwatch could be used as a phone and a calendar, or even a GPS system to prevent the wearer from becoming lost, especially if tracked by a caregiver.
- Instead of restraints and wheelchairs, nursing homes should offer more opportunities for exercise. Small plots where patients can garden or care for plants can provide an active outdoor exercise. Indoor volleyball and miniature golf are offered at some day-care facilities. Stretching and yoga are excellent exercises to improve flexibility and reduce stress through calm relaxation. Meditation, as stated previously, can even improve cognitive processing.
- Allowing pets in some instances can offer companionship and comfort. The interaction with a pet may serve as a stimulus for the brain. One man with AD who had lost almost all of his speech recovers some of it when he is with his dog, as shown on a YouTube video, "My Dad with Our Dog," that has attracted almost six million visitors.
- Blank walls and washable finger paints or other preschool activities for creativity may be a good model. Pottery and

workshops in woodcraft can be taught at day-care facilities along with crafts for making holiday decorations.

- Music can be either soothing or bring memories of a happier period of youth. Drumming can be a physical outlet of expression. Some centers, like the Tidewater Arts Outreach program in Taos, have choirs for their residents. My mother's happiest moments during her five years living in memory care were spent singing along with the talented activity director while he played the keyboard. The long-remembered lyrics transported her back decades.

On my last visit to see my mother in the long-term care unit, I was impressed to see a full staff of aides, a social worker, rehabilitation therapists, and, surprisingly, an activity director, in addition to the nurses present around the clock. Although my mother still slept most of the time in her wheelchair during the day, other, more active, patients were treated to parties for every holiday (including being dressed in costumes for Halloween) and field trips to some of the nearby casinos and to the wax museum. Large colored photos of each of these activities lined one of the hallways, and famous Norman Rockwell prints of an earlier era were displayed in other halls, so that in spite of the hospital environment, a more cheerful look pervaded the long-term care unit and the individual rooms, each with decorative wallpaper and colorful textile valances over the windows.

In Mother's room, my brother or his wife had hung family photos on the walls just as they had done in the other rooms where she lived. This time they'd also brought a radio/compact disc player with a Benny Goodman CD inside. But like my father eight years earlier, Mom didn't want to hear songs anymore. Even music had lost its charm.


On my recent visit in July 2014, Mom was thinner and her left eyelid drooped. Since that was her good eye, I wasn't sure she could see me at first when the attendant wheeled her into the lunchroom.

I watched as with a little help she fed herself a hearty lunch. Then I sat with her in the otherwise empty television room while she dozed after eating. Finally, back in her room, we could begin to visit; she was still in her wheelchair, not on her bed. Mom listened closely as I reminisced with her about things she used to do, such as give us a piece of chocolate on Sunday afternoons. Now I fed her pieces of chocolate from the box I had brought to give her. Many of the words she attempted to say did not come out right, but she did speak one sentence quite clearly.

She said, "I thought we were going home now."


Feelings—desires, hopes—don't go away. Our minds are filled with many states besides memory—emotions, beliefs, desires, wishes, intentions, and creativity. Someday we must recognize that one's personhood doesn't need to be defined solely by one's ability to remember. Someday there will be new ways of helping the elderly with Alzheimer's and other diseases, ways that focus on the person inside instead of on the illness, based on a model that treats each of them with respect, attention, and dignity.

Because the title of this book is from the poem *Do Not Go Gently* by Dylan Thomas, ending with another excerpt from poetry seems appropriate. These lines, from Robert Browning, are more optimistic:

> Grow old along with me!
> The best is yet to be,
> The last of life, for which the first was made. . .

When we are able to fight back successfully against Alzheimer's disease and other dementias, we can make the last of life a time of happiness instead of ending by not going gently.

# ACKNOWLEDGMENTS

My greatest thanks go to my husband, Ed, for his unflagging support and encouragement, and for the number of times he patiently read each draft of every chapter, always offering his excellent advice and often finding errors. For her ideas and contributions to the first chapter, I want to thank my daughter Karen Kirkbride. My son Mark Hanley gave me editorial and content advice. I'm fortunate to count two professional writers among my good friends, Deanne Mincer and Marjorie Ford, who guided and encouraged me at the beginning. Several other friends who read an early draft of the first chapters urged me to express my feelings openly, and my thanks go to Judy McCormick, Stephanie Buch, Judy Jackson-Coebergh, and Pat Critzer. Those who read the completed first draft deserve a medal for reviewing what was still a half-finished manuscript, but who nevertheless gave me positive feedback to continue: especially Jerrine Barrett, Gerry Meloy, and Marc Saunders. For the intrepid readers who offered editorial comments and suggestions for that first draft, I'm especially grateful to MaryAnn Saunders, Vera Berg, Barrie Fairley, M.D., and retired Judge James Barton Phelps. Thank you also to the wonderful editorial team who helped so much.

The Alzheimer's Association Education and Referral (ADEAR) Center offers reliable information for families and professionals at www.nia.nih.gov/Alzheimers.

The Alzheimer Research Forum is at www.alzforum.org.

And, of course, the Alzheimer's Association at www.alz.org is the gateway to multiple services, support, and education.

Each of these sites is a source for excellent, helpful information and up-to-date news.

# CHAPTER NOTES

Preface

[1] R. Hitt et al., "Centenarians: the older you get, the younger you have been," *Lancet* 354 (1999): 652.

[2] Peter V. Rabins, MD, MPH, *The Johns Hopkins White Papers: Memory* (New York: Remedy Health Media, 2013), 30.

Chapter 2 Lonely

[3] Carla Persissinotto, MD, MHS, Irena Stiljacic, MA, and Kenneth Covinsky, MD, MPH, "Loneliness in Older Persons: A predictor of functional decline and death," *JAMA Internal Medicine* 172 (2012): 1078–-84.

[4] Cathy Alessi, MD, quoted in Caroline Grannan, *Caregiver*, my.webmd.com/ content/pages/5/4041_129.htm.

[5] DE Barnes et al., "Mid-life versus late-life depressive symptoms and risk of dementia," *Archives of General Psychiatry* 69 (2012): 493–98.Mid-life versus late-life depressive symptoms and risk of dementia: Differential effects for Alzheimer's disease and vascular dementia

Chapter 3 Lacking

[6] Peter V. Rabins, MD, MPH, ed., *Johns Hopkins Medicine: Alzheimer's Outlook 2013* (New York: Remedy Health Media, 2013), 6.

[7] Rabins, *Memory*, 22–23; 62–63.

[8] T. Psaltopoulou et al., "Mediterranean diet, stroke, cognitive impairment, and depression: A meta-analysis," *Annals of Neurology* 74 (October 2013): 580–91, doi: 10.1002/ana.23944.
Soni Lourida et al., "Mediterranean diet, cognitive function, and dementia: a systematic review," *Epidemiology* 24 (2013): 479–89.

[9] EE Devore, JH Kang, MM Breteler, F Goldstein, "Dietary intakes of berries and flavonoids in relation to cognitive decline," *Annals of Neurology* 72 (2012): 135–43.

[10] F. Yang et al., "Curcumin Inhibits Formation of Amyloid Oligomers and Fibrils, Binds Plaques, and Reduces Amyloid in Vivo," *Journal of Biological Chemistry* 280 (2005): 5892-5901.

[11] Michael Ramscar, PhD, et al., "The Myth of Cognitive Decline: Non-Linear Dynamics of Lifelong Learning," *Topics in Cognitive Science* 6 (January 2014), doi: 10.1111/tops.12078.

Chapter 4 Locked In

[12] Cindy Barton, RN, MSN, "Hospitalization," paper presented at UCSF Memory and Aging Center Research Event, San Francisco, March 18, 2014.

[13] Sam Gandy, MD, PhD, quoted in Steven Reinberg, "Anemia Might Raise Dementia Risk, Study Suggests," http://consumer.healthday.com/senior-citizen-information-31/misc-aging-news-10/low-iron-might-raise-dementia-risk-study-suggests-678791.html

[14] Rabins, *Memory*, 32–38.

[15] Gary Small, MD, et al., "Prediction of Cognitive Decline by Positron Emission Tomography of Brain Amyloid and Tau," *Archives of Neurology* 69 (2012): 215, accessed February 15, 2012, doi: 10.1001/archneurol.2011.559.

[16] Claudia H. Kawas, MD, "The Oldest Old: Findings from the 90+ Study," in *Alzheimer's Outlook 2013*, ed. Rabins, 26.

[17] Barry Reisberg, MD, et al., "The global deterioration scale for assessment of primary degenerative dementia," *American Journal of Psychiatry* 139 (September 1982): 1136–39, www.ncbi.nim.gov/pubmed/7114305.

[18] Rabins, *Memory*, 29.

Chapter 5 Lights Out

[19] Shin Yeu Ong et al., "Visual impairment, age-related eye diseases, and cognitive function: The Singapore Malay Eye Study," *Archives of Ophthalmology* 130 (July 2012): 895–900, doi: 10.1001/archophthalmol.2012.152.

[20] Maya Koronyo-Hamaoui et al., "Identification of amyloid plaques in retinas from Alzheimer's patients and noninvasive in vivo optical imaging of retinal plaques in a mouse model," *NeuroImage* 54 (January 2011): s204–17, published online June 13, 2010, accessed August 23, 2013, doi: 10.1016/j.neuroimage.2010.06.020.

Chapter 6 Letting Go

[21] Leonard Berg, MD, et al., "Relation of Histologic Markers to Dementia Severity, Age, Sex, and Apolipoprotein E Genotype," *Archives of Neurology,* 55 (1998): 326–35, doi: 10.1001/archneur.55.3.326.

[22] William James, *The Varieties of Religious Experience.* New York: The New American Library, 1958.

[23] Timothy Ferris, "Mind Games," *Image,* February 2, 1992, 22–26.

[24] Eric Kandel, MD, "The New Science of Mind," *The New York Times,* September 8, 2013.

[25] Jean-Dominique Bauby, *The Diving Bell and the Butterfly.* New York: Knopf Doubleday Publishing Group, 2007.

[26] Oliver Sacks, *Awakenings.* New York: Vintage Books, 1990.

[27] Bryan D. James, PhD, et al., "Contribution of Alzheimer disease to mortality in the United States," *Neurology* 82 (March 2014): 1045–50, published online before print March 5, 2014, doi: 10.1212/ WNL.0000000000000240Neurology.

Chapter 7 Latent Gene
[28] Alzheimer's Association, *2014 Alzheimer's Disease Facts and Figures,* March 19, 2014.

[29] Pierre N. Tariot, MD, "The Alzheimer's Prevention Initiative Study," *Alzheimer's Outlook 2013*, ed. Rabins, 48.

[30] Rabins, *Memory*, 43–44.

[31] Gary Small, MD, quoted in Jean Carper, *100 Simple Things You Can Do to Prevent Alzheimer's* (New York: Little, Brown, 2011).

[32] Gary Small, MD, quoted in Lisa Davis, "Is My Memory Normal?" *AARP*, June/July 2013, 47.

[33] Gretchen Reynolds, "How Exercise May Keep Alzheimer's at Bay," *Well Blog, New York Times,* January 18, 2012, well.blogs.newyork.times.com/2008/07/15/.

[34] Laura L. Carstensen, quoted in Margery D. Rosen, "Get Moving for a Healthy Brain," *AARP*, September 2013, 12.

[35] Kirk Erickson quoted in M. Rosen, *AARP, 13*.

[36] John Medina quoted in M. Rosen, *AARP, 12*.

[37] Rabins, *Memory*, 17.

[38] E. Luders et al., "The unique brain anatomy of meditation practitioners: alterations in cortical gyrification," *Frontiers in Human Neuroscience* 6 (February 2012), doi: 10.3389/fnhum.2012.0034.e collection 2012.

[39] JV Pottala, K. Jaffe et al., "Higher RBC EPA+ DHA corresponds with larger total brain and hippocampal volumes: WHIMS-MRI Study," Neurology (January 2014), doi:10.1212/WNL.0000000000000080.

[40] Vencenzo Solfrizzi et al., "Alcohol consumption, mild cognitive impairment, and progression to dementia," Neurology 68 (2007): 2.

[41] KJ Mulkamal et al., "Prospective study of alcohol consumption and risk of dementia in older adults," JAMA (2003): 1405–13.

[42] Rabins, Memory, 34.

[43] Farzaneh Sorond et al., "Neurovascular coupling, cerebral white matter integrity, and response to cocoa in older people," Neurology, published ahead of print August 7, 2013, doi: 10.1212/WNL.0b013e3182a351aa.

[44] L. Kerti et al., "Higher glucose levels associated with lower memory and reduced hippocampal microstructure," Neurology (2013): 1746–52.

[45] Rabins, Memory, 25.

[46] Benedict Carey, "The Older Mind May Just Be a Fuller Mind," The New York Times, January 27, 2014.

[47] "The Conversation Project," Institute for Healthcare Improvement, www.ihi.org/offerings/initiatives/ ConversationProject/Pages/default.aspx.

[48] "The Five Wishes," Aging with Dignity, accessed June13, 2014, agingwithdignity.org/index.php

## Chapter 8 Looking Ahead

[49] Susan Collins interviewed by Michael Hedges, "Conversation With," *AARP Bulletin/Real Possibilities,* December 2013, 8.

[50] William Fisher and Lennart Mucke, "Open Forum on Alzheimer's Disease: Research Targets Treatments," *San Francisco Chronicle,* August 2013.

[51] John C. Morris, MD, "The DIAN Study," in *Alzheimer's Outlook 2013,* ed. Rabins, 40–45.

[52] "Alzheimer's Disease: Big federal grant shifts research to prevention," *The New York Times (reprint in San Francisco Chronicle,* September 20, 2013).

[53] Lennart Mucke, MD quoted in Erin Allday, "New Ideas in Search for a Cure," *San Francisco Chronicle,* November 20, 2013.

[54] Eric Kandel, MD quoted in "Health: Memory loss due to aging found to be distinct from Alzheimer's," AP report in *San Francisco Chronicle,* August 29, 2013.

[55] Erin Allday, "Alzheimer's Disease: Tau research," *San Francisco Chronicle,* September 4, 2013.

[56] Dena Dubal et al., "Life Extension Factor Enhances Cognition," *Cell Reports 7* (May 2014) 1065-76, accessed May 13, 2014, doi: 0.1016/j.celrep.2014.03.076.

[57] Ron Winslow, "New Research Path for Memory Loss," *U.S. News,* May 5, 2014.

[58] Michelle Castillo "11 new gene variants linked to Alzheimer's disease," CBS News, October 28, 2013, www.cbsnews.com/8301_204_162_57609581/ (site discontinued).

[59] Erin Allday, "Health: Protein linked to brain disorders," *San Francisco Chronicle*, August 21, 2013.

[60] Erin Allday, "Reduced protein may make brain vulnerable," *San Francisco Chronicle*, September 18, 2013.

[61] Matthew Blurton-Jones, PhD, "Examining the Effects of Neural Stem Cell Transplantation in Transgenic Models of Alzheimer's," paper presented at University of California Irvine colloquium, February 14, 2014.

[62] Stephanie M. Lee, "Memory Loss: Small structure in brain may hold key," *San Francisco Chronicle*, September 25, 2013.

[63] Suzanne Craft et al., "Intranasal Insulin Therapy for Alzheimer's Dementia and Amnestic Mild Cognitive Impairment, *Archives of Neurology* 69 (January 2012): 29-38, accessed February 3, 2014, doi: 10.100/archneurol 2011.233.

[64] Lucas Restrepo et al., "High Accuracy of a Microarray-Based Blood Test for Alzheimer's Disease," *Neurology* 82 (2014): 10.

[65] Stephanie M. Lee, "Electronics of the body," *San Francisco Chronicle*, May 26, 2014.

[66] Tena Alonzo quoted in Rebecca Mead, "The Sense of an Ending," *The New Yorker*, May 20, 2013.

# AUTHOR BIO

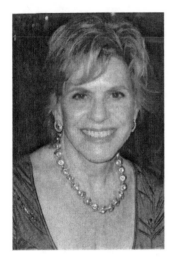

Constance L. Vincent, PhD, a psychologist with expertise on aging, graduated Phi Beta Kappa from Ohio University before earning her doctorate from UC Irvine. She taught developmental psychology first as an associate professor at Chapman University and later at Santa Clara University.

As the daughter of a father who suffered from dementia and a mother who has Alzheimer's, Dr. Vincent knows she too carries the potential for these diseases. A long-distance caregiver for her mother, she serves her local community by presenting for the Alzheimer's Speakers Bureau and supporting senior programs through Peninsula Volunteers. Committed to sharing her knowledge about new approaches for early prevention, Dr. Vincent wrote *Not Going Gently* to educate and encourage readers through her personal story and scientific research.

Dr. Vincent and her husband live in Menlo Park, California. They enjoy traveling, attending the opera and symphony, and participating in book clubs. They have a son, four daughters, and twelve grandchildren.

CPSIA information can be obtained at www.ICGtesting.com
Printed in the USA
LVOW07s1742221015

459348LV00009B/86/P

9 781499 512595